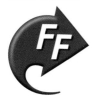

Fast Facts

Fast Facts:
Hyperlipidemia

Fifth edition

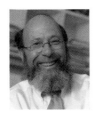

Allan Sniderman MD FRCP(C)
Edwards Professor of Cardiology
and Professor of Medicine
McGill University
Montreal, Canada

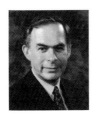

Paul Durrington MD FRCP FRCPath FMedSci
Professor of Medicine
Cardiovascular Research Group
School of Clinical and Laboratory Science
University of Manchester, UK

D1225879

Declaration of Independ
This book is as balanced an... ...
Ideas for improvement are always welcome: feedback@fastfacts.com

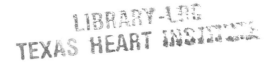
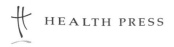

HEALTH PRESS

Fast Facts: Hyperlipidemia
First published 2000
Second edition 2002
Third edition 2005
Fourth edition April 2008, reprinted 2008
Fifth edition June 2010

Health Press Limited, Elizabeth House, Queen Street, Abingdon,
Oxford OX14 3LN, UK
Tel: +44 (0)1235 523233
Fax: +44 (0)1235 523238

Book orders can be placed by telephone or via the website.
For regional distributors or to order via the website, please go to:
www.fastfacts.com

For telephone orders, please call +44 (0)1752 202301 (UK and Europe),
1 800 247 6553 (USA, toll free), +1 419 281 1802 (Americas)
or +61 (0)2 9698 7755 (Asia–Pacific).

Fast Facts is a trademark of Health Press Limited.

The publisher and the authors have made every effort to ensure the accuracy of this
book, but cannot accept responsibility for any errors or omissions.

For all drugs, please consult the product labeling approved in your country for
prescribing information.

A CIP record for this title is available from the British Library.

ISBN 978-1-905832-63-7

Author: Sniderman, A (Allan)
Fast Facts: Hyperlipidemia/
Allan Sniderman, Paul Durrington

Medical illustrations by Dee McLean, London, UK.
Typesetting and page layout by Zed, Oxford, UK.
Printed by Latimer Trend & Company Ltd, Plymouth, UK.

Text printed on biodegradable and recyclable paper
manufactured using elemental chlorine free (ECF)
wood pulp from well-managed forests.

FSC
Mixed Sources
Product group from well-managed
forests and other controlled sources
Cert no. SGS-COC-005493
www.fsc.org
© 1996 Forest Stewardship Council

Glossary

Android obesity: male-pattern obesity, characterized by increased accumulation of abdominal adipose tissue

ApoAI: apolipoprotein AI, the major apolipoprotein in HDL

ApoB$_{48}$: gut apolipoprotein B (its molecular weight is 48% of that of apoB$_{100}$)

ApoB$_{100}$: hepatic apolipoprotein B

Apolipoproteins: structural proteins, often containing receptor-binding sites

ARH: autosomal recessive hypercholesterolemia

ATPIII: Third Adult Treatment Panel of the NCEP (USA)

β-VLDL: chylomicron remnants and intermediate-density lipoprotein

CETP: cholesteryl ester transfer protein, which catalyzes transfer of cholesterol from HDL to circulating triglyceride-rich lipoproteins, and from LDL back to VLDL

CHD: coronary heart disease

Cholesteryl ester: esterified cholesterol, which is more hydrophobic than free cholesterol

CVD: cardiovascular disease

FCHL: familial combined hyperlipidemia

FDB: familial defective apoB

FH: familial hypercholesterolemia

Foam cell: a cell, usually a macrophage, the cytoplasm of which has become loaded with cholesterol

Gynoid obesity: female-pattern obesity, characterized by increased depots in the buttocks and other peripheral sites

HDL: high-density lipoprotein

HyperapoB: hyperapobetalipoproteinemia, raised apoB in the absence of a raised LDL cholesterol level

IDL: intermediate-density lipoprotein

LCAT: lecithin–cholesterol acyl transferase, which catalyzes the esterification of free cholesterol

LDL: low-density lipoprotein

Lipemia retinalis: pallor of the optic fundus and white appearance of the retinal veins and arteries caused by extremely high levels of circulating chylomicrons

Lp(a): lipoprotein (a), an LDL-like particle that contains apolipoprotein (a) in addition to apoB

LPL: lipoprotein lipase, an enzyme which breaks down triglycerides into fatty acids

LpX: lipoprotein X, an abnormal lipoprotein present in plasma in obstructive jaundice

LRP: LDL receptor-related protein

NASH: non-alcohol hepatic steatohepatitis (also known as non-alcoholic fatty liver disease)

NCEP: National Cholesterol Education Program (USA)

NEFA: non-esterified fatty acids

PCSK9: proprotein convertase subtilisin/kexin type 9

SCORE: Systematic Coronary Risk Evaluation

Small, dense LDL: cholesterol-depleted LDL

TSH: thyroid-stimulating hormone

VLDL: very-low-density lipoprotein

A note on conversion of units
So that values will accord more closely with those chosen by various consensus groups, we have sometimes used a factor of 40, rather than the more precise 38.6, to convert between mmol/L and mg/dL as units of cholesterol concentration. Similarly, a conversion factor of 90 has been used for triglycerides. Converted values are given to two significant figures.

Introduction

This edition, like earlier ones, is directed at a broad range of healthcare professionals, from primary care physicians to specialists. Our objective is to present a crisp and accurate summary of the field. In particular, we want to outline a coherent pathophysiological structure on which the physician can build a sound diagnostic and clinical approach.

Vascular disease is not beaten, but it is retreating, and it is therefore critical that we apply as rapidly as possible the major clinical and scientific advances that have occurred. Guidelines are one way to speed implementation – they are invaluable for guiding clinical practice – but they do not substitute for clear knowledge of the issues at stake.

That is why we have tried to provide a text that interprets clinical trial evidence in the context of pathogenesis and gives practical solutions to routine problems encountered in the clinical management of hyperlipidemias.

In this fifth edition, the importance of considering lipoprotein particles, not just their lipids, is addressed, with reference to the latest evidence. The emphasis on including apoB as a core clinical parameter distinguishes our presentation of the issues from most others. While we may be a bit ahead, we are not alone. The approach we advocate to assessment of the adequacy of low-density lipoprotein lowering therapy corresponds to that in the recent Consensus Statements issued by the American Diabetes Association, the American College of Cardiology and the American Association for Clinical Chemistry.

1 Lipids and lipoproteins – structure and physiology

Lipoprotein particles are macromolecular complexes of lipids – cholesterol, cholesteryl ester, triglycerides and phospholipids – and proteins (Figure 1.1). The outer membrane of all lipoprotein particles is

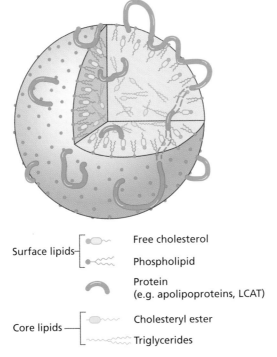

Surface lipids
- Free cholesterol
- Phospholipid
- Protein (e.g. apolipoproteins, LCAT)

Core lipids
- Cholesteryl ester
- Triglycerides

Figure 1.1 The structure of a lipoprotein. The most hydrophobic components (the triglycerides and cholesteryl esters) form a central droplet, which is surrounded by the more polar components (free cholesterol, proteins and phospholipids). Proteins are arranged with their hydrophobic sequences inside the particle and their hydrophilic regions oriented towards the aqueous environment. The polar groups of cholesterol and phospholipids also point outwards, away from the hydrophobic core. LCAT, lecithin–cholesterol acyl transferase.

a phospholipid monolayer. The apolipoproteins are the protein components – they differ in function and in whether or not they can leave one lipoprotein particle for another.

The four types of lipoprotein particle

Chylomicrons and very-low-density lipoproteins (VLDL) are the two triglyceride-rich lipoproteins, whereas low- and high-density lipoproteins (LDL and HDL, respectively) are the two cholesterol-rich lipoproteins. All four are illustrated in Figure 1.2.

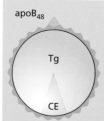

Chylomicrons are produced by the gut after the digestion of fat. Of the four lipoproteins, they are the richest in triglycerides (Tg). The triglycerides are removed from the chylomicrons either for energy in muscle or for storage in adipose tissue, and the remnants circulate until they are taken up by the liver. Each chylomicron also contains many different apolipoproteins, including one molecule of apoB$_{48}$ and others such as apoE and apoCII.

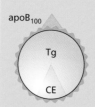

Very-low-density lipoprotein (VLDL) particles are produced by the liver. They contain more triglyceride than cholesterol. As the triglycerides are removed for energy or storage, the VLDL remnants continue to circulate as low-density lipoprotein (LDL) particles. Each VLDL particle contains apoE, one molecule of apoB$_{100}$ (another form of apoB), and several other apolipoproteins.

LDL particles are composed primarily of cholesterol – as cholesteryl ester (CE) or free cholesterol – and some triglycerides. About 70% of serum cholesterol is carried by these lipoproteins, so the concentration of total serum cholesterol largely reflects the LDL cholesterol concentration. LDL particles are remnants of VLDL particles, but they contain only a single apolipoprotein, apoB$_{100}$.

High-density lipoprotein (HDL) particles contain one-fifth to one-third serum cholesterol. They transport excess cholesterol from the tissues to the liver and to other lipoprotein particles, such as VLDL. This process is known as reverse cholesterol transport. HDL particles also contain apolipoproteins, including apoAI and often apoAII.

Figure 1.2 Four types of lipoprotein particle.

Chylomicrons and VLDL. Chylomicrons are much larger than VLDL particles, and correspondingly contain much more triglyceride per particle. Chylomicrons transport dietary triglyceride from the intestine whereas VLDL particles transport triglyceride from the liver.

LDL. Most of the cholesterol present in plasma is found in LDL particles. LDL particles, however, vary in size with the amount of cholesterol they contain (Figure 1.3). The smaller particles contain less cholesterol and, as lipids are less dense than proteins, are denser than the larger particles. Particle for particle, the smaller, denser LDLs are at least as atherogenic as the larger, more buoyant LDLs.

The process by which small, dense LDL particles are formed is illustrated in Figure 1.4. Step 1 occurs when cholesteryl ester transfer protein (CETP) allows cholesteryl ester from an LDL particle to be exchanged for triglyceride from VLDL. Step 2 occurs when the triglyceride is removed via hydrolysis by hepatic lipase to produce a smaller, denser LDL particle.

HDL particles play a critical role in the transport of cholesterol from peripheral cells to the liver. Low levels of HDL are associated with an

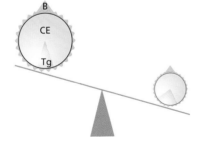

↑ Entry rate into artery wall

↑ Oxidation

↑ Secretion of PAI-1

↓ EDRF

↑ Thromboxane

↑ Sticking to glycosaminoglycans

Figure 1.3 Small, dense low-density lipoprotein (LDL) particles are at least as atherogenic as the larger, more buoyant LDL particles, even though they contain less cholesterol. Based on in-vitro studies, they enter the vessel wall more readily, they oxidize more readily and they are more thrombogenic. B, apoB; CE, cholesteryl ester; Tg, triglyceride; PAI-1, plasminogen activator inhibitor type 1; EDRF, endothelium-derived relaxing factor.

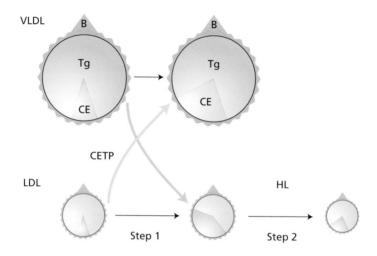

Figure 1.4 How small, dense low-density lipoprotein (LDL) particles are formed in plasma: LDL remodeling by cholesterol–triglyceride (Tg) exchange and hydrolysis. B, apoB; CE, cholesteryl ester; CETP, cholesteryl ester transfer protein; HL, hepatic lipase; VLDL, very-low-density lipoprotein.

increased risk of coronary heart disease (CHD), a relationship which is particularly prominent when LDL levels – indicated by either LDL cholesterol or apoB concentration (see later) – are elevated. HDL levels are generally low in patients with hypertriglyceridemia by virtue of the same remodeling mechanisms that are responsible for the generation of small, dense LDL particles. HDL levels can be quantified by measuring HDL cholesterol or by measuring the level of apolipoprotein AI (apoAI), the major apolipoprotein in HDL. More than one apoAI molecule can be present in each HDL particle so the serum apoAI level does not necessarily reflect the HDL particle concentration. Nevertheless, there is now evidence that serum apoAI may be more informative of cardiovascular risk than levels of HDL cholesterol.

Apolipoprotein B

The most important apolipoprotein for our purposes is the B apolipoprotein (apoB), of which there are two forms: $apoB_{100}$ and

$apoB_{48}$. Each VLDL and LDL particle contains one molecule of $apoB_{100}$, whereas each chylomicron particle contains one molecule of $apoB_{48}$, which is a truncated version of $apoB_{100}$. Both $apoB_{100}$ and $apoB_{48}$ remain with their respective particles until the particles are removed from the circulation. Not only does $apoB_{100}$ provide structural integrity to the particle, but also a critical region binds to the LDL receptor, and it is this interaction which results in the irreversible removal of LDL from plasma.

ApoB particles are atherogenic. Because there is one apoB molecule per particle, serum apoB gives an exact measure of the number of atherogenic particles in plasma; further, because chylomicron particles never constitute more than 1% and VLDL particles account for less than 10% of lipoprotein particles, the level of apoB gives a good estimate of LDL particle number. Moreover, because chylomicrons are so few in number, even postprandially, patients do not have to be fasting when plasma apoB level is measured, a major advantage in clinical practice.

Lipid and lipoprotein metabolism

Biological role of triglycerides and fatty acids. Triglyceride is a major source of energy and is stored in adipose tissue subcutaneously where it insulates against heat loss, and internally where it protects viscera against physical damage. It can be transported either as triglyceride in lipoproteins or, after hydrolysis by a lipase (lipolysis), as its constituent fatty acids. The latter are termed non-esterified fatty acids (NEFA) and circulate bound to albumin.

Triglyceride transport and storage. Triglycerides are an almost ideal form of energy storage and consequently are, far and away, the major form in which we store energy. Almost one-fifth of the total mass of a lean, 70 kg adult man is made up of triglyceride in adipose tissue. If oxidized, this would yield 570 000 kilojoules – roughly enough energy to survive total starvation for 3 months. Certainly in the long term, triglycerides are a far more important source of energy than glycogen, the total store of which would yield fewer than 4200 kilojoules.

Adipose tissue is the major site of triglyceride storage, and the adipose cell appears morphologically to be no more than a rim of cytoplasm around a large droplet of triglyceride. These cells, however, are much more active metabolically than their structure suggests. Not only is the rate at which they take up and release fatty acids tightly regulated, but they also synthesize and secrete a wide variety of bioactive molecules.

Visceral adipose tissue produces hormones, such as resistin and retinol-binding protein 4, and inflammatory cytokines, like tumor necrosis factor X and interleukin 6, which cause insulin resistance and thus increase the tendency to release NEFA. When there is central obesity, these processes are important in the genesis of metabolic syndrome and type 2 diabetes (see Chapter 7).

The metabolism of chylomicrons and VLDL is illustrated in Figure 1.5. Dietary triglycerides undergo digestion in the gut to fatty acids and monoglycerides. These are absorbed into the enterocytes, resynthesized into triglycerides and packaged into chylomicrons, and then enter the circulation for transport to the tissues. Fat absorption is generally complete within a few hours, and during this time plasma triglyceride levels increase, though the degree to which they do so is very modest in healthy people. In some people, however, triglyceride clearance is delayed, and postprandial hypertriglyceridemia is an important clinical finding.

At the capillary endothelial surfaces in adipose tissue and in cardiac and skeletal muscle, the enzyme lipoprotein lipase (LPL) rapidly breaks down the triglycerides within chylomicrons, releasing large amounts of fatty acids. Muscle is extremely effective at taking up these fatty acids, most of which are almost immediately oxidized for energy. Surprisingly, adipose tissue is less effective, with only about two-thirds of the fatty acids that are released being taken up on average; the rest are bound to albumin and then circulate in plasma as NEFA.

After encountering LPL, chylomicrons become relatively triglyceride-poor and cholesterol-rich remnants. Normally, these remnants are rapidly removed by the liver via receptor-mediated mechanisms that involve a multifunctional receptor, the LDL receptor-related protein (LRP),

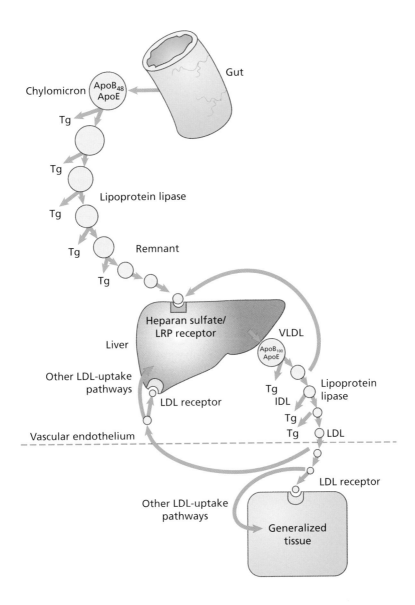

Figure 1.5 Metabolism of chylomicrons, very-low-density lipoprotein (VLDL) and low-density lipoprotein (LDL). Triglyceride (Tg) is released from chylomicrons and VLDL as glycerol, monoglycerides and non-esterified fatty acids. Apo, apolipoprotein; IDL, intermediate-density lipoprotein; LRP, LDL receptor-related protein.

13

and the proteoglycan heparan sulfate, on the surface of hepatocytes. The chylomicron remnant ligand for this receptor is apoE, which it acquires during its time in the circulation (see Chapter 6). Accumulation of chylomicron remnants in the plasma is extremely atherogenic.

The fatty acids taken up by adipocytes are reformed into triglycerides. During fasting, when energy is required elsewhere, the adipose tissue triglycerides are hydrolyzed by an intracellular enzyme, hormone-sensitive lipase, releasing fatty acids from adipose tissue. When large amounts of energy are required rapidly, as during exercise, the activity of hormone-sensitive lipase is increased by catecholamines, releasing additional fatty acids as metabolic fuel.

VLDL particles undergo the same metabolic fate as chylomicrons, with one important difference. Just as with chylomicrons, the triglyceride within them is broken down by LPL on the capillary endothelium of muscle and adipose tissue, and fatty acids are released which may be taken up by adipose tissue or muscle or circulate as NEFA. However, whereas the chylomicron remnants produced are, in general, rapidly removed from the circulation by the liver, most VLDL particles become converted to LDL particles.

LDL particles persist in plasma nine times longer than VLDL particles. That is why there are always nine times more LDL than VLDL particles. In addition, LDL particles are much smaller than VLDL particles. Therefore, they can pass through the vascular endothelium much more easily. Those two facts explain why LDL is more directly important in atherogenesis than VLDL.

Another point to note is that the proportion of fatty acids taken up by adipose tissue varies. This is due in part to variation in the efficiency of the mechanism for trapping fatty acids in the adipose tissue. If fewer fatty acids are taken up by adipose tissue, more will remain in the circulation, and therefore more will be carried to the liver. The increased flux of fatty acids to the liver results in increased hepatic triglyceride synthesis and secretion, which is accompanied by increased secretion of VLDL particles. The increased secretion of VLDL particles results in increased production of LDL particles.

Biological role of cholesterol

Cholesterol is an essential component of all cell membranes, where it occupies spaces between the molecules of the phospholipid bilayer, reducing its fluidity. Cholesterol is the precursor for bile acid, steroid hormone and vitamin D synthesis.

Cholesterol metabolism and transport in lipoproteins. Typically, the daily cholesterol intake is 200–500 mg/day, whereas the total dietary fat intake is 80–100 g/day. Furthermore, cholesterol absorption from the gut is incomplete, with only 30–60% actually entering the body. Chylomicrons then transport this cholesterol of exogenous origin from the intestine to the liver, where the chylomicron remnants are taken up (Figure 1.5).

In total, the body synthesizes at least as much cholesterol as it absorbs. Although all the cells in the body can synthesize cholesterol, most cholesterol synthesis is centralized in the liver, the gut and the central nervous system. This is because LDL is small enough to cross the vascular endothelium of all tissues other than the central nervous system (blood–brain barrier). As a consequence, most cells are in contact with LDL and can synthesize LDL receptors which bind to $apoB_{100}$, permitting LDL entry into the cell to supply cholesterol.

Cholesterol biosynthesis is extremely complex. However, a key regulatory step occurs early in the pathway, at the point where 3-hydroxy-3-methylglutaryl coenzyme A (HMG-CoA) is converted to mevalonic acid. The enzyme responsible, HMG-CoA reductase, can be inhibited by a variety of factors, the most important of which for clinical purposes are the statin drugs (otherwise known as HMG-CoA reductase inhibitors).

The liver is the central clearing house for cholesterol, with several ways in and out. When cytoplasmic cholesterol levels decline in the liver (for example, with statin treatment; when cholesterol re-absorption from the small intestine is decreased by cholesterol absorption inhibitors, such as plant sterol or stanol esters added to food products, or the drug ezetimibe; or when fasting), hepatic LDL-receptor expression increases. This accelerates the rate of hepatic clearance of LDL from the circulation, lowering LDL cholesterol. Only hepatocytes can eliminate cholesterol from the body. They break it down to bile acids and also secrete it dissolved with bile acids in the bile destined to enter the small intestine. This is the major route by which cholesterol can leave the body. Of the total reaching the small intestine, however, a variable but important amount is reabsorbed, resulting in enterohepatic cholesterol cycling. Interruption of this cycle by cholesterol absorption inhibition, e.g. with ezetimibe, or sequestration of bile acids necessary for producing cholesterol-containing micelles small enough for efficient cholesterol absorption, e.g. colesevelam, lowers serum cholesterol (see previous page).

Hepatic secretion of cholesterol, mostly as VLDL, exceeds the requirement of tissues. This excess cholesterol must return to the liver via either LDL or HDL particles if it is not to accumulate in the tissues. However, this is a largely futile and potentially dangerous (atherosclerotic) cycle.

HDL and reverse cholesterol transport

HDL plays a critical role in the transport of cholesterol from peripheral tissues back to the liver (Figure 1.6). Small HDL particles receive free cholesterol after it leaves the cells of the peripheral tissues via an ATP-binding cassette transporter. The free cholesterol is then mostly converted to cholesteryl ester located on HDL by the enzyme lecithin–cholesterol acyl transferase. The cholesteryl ester formed is much more hydrophobic than free cholesterol and so can be tightly packed within the core of the HDL particle, allowing HDL to pick up more cholesterol. Cholesterol can be returned directly to the liver from HDL by the class B type I hepatic scavenger receptor which, unlike the other receptors discussed so far, removes cholesteryl ester and free cholesterol from HDL without catabolizing the HDL particles, which are returned to the circulation depleted of cholesterol. Alternatively, cholesteryl ester can be transferred out of HDL in the circulation to VLDL in exchange for triglyceride, a process mediated by CETP. The cholesteryl ester can then be returned to the liver in VLDL and/or LDL particles. It can also, of course, be delivered back to the tissues in the same lipoproteins, making it difficult to predict whether CETP is potentially atherogenic or anti-atherogenic. Recently, torcetrapib, the first of the CETP inhibitors, was withdrawn

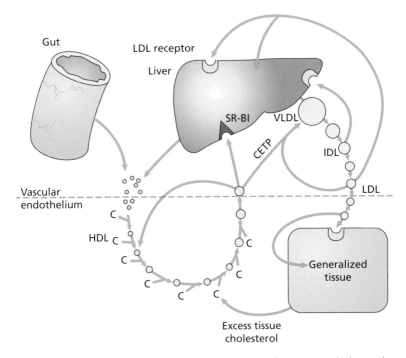

Figure 1.6 High-density lipoprotein (HDL) is involved in reverse cholesterol transport. Excess cholesterol (C) from the tissues is released to HDL and is then delivered to either the liver or very-low-density lipoprotein (VLDL) in a process mediated by cholesteryl ester transfer protein (CETP). Some cholesteryl ester can be returned to the liver via low-density lipoprotein (LDL), but it can also find its way back to the tissues. IDL, intermediate-density lipoprotein; SR-BI, scavenger receptor class B type I.

from further development because of increased adverse cardiovascular events. Future trials will reveal whether the effect was specific to this compound and whether other members of this class show benefit.

Epidemiological studies have repeatedly shown that both LDL and HDL are major determinants of the risk of vascular disease. Risk increases as LDL increases. However, at any level of LDL, risk is also determined by HDL. Low levels of HDL are associated with an increased risk of CHD, and HDL is believed to play a major protective role against atherosclerosis. This could occur in many ways. One is by promoting the transfer of cholesterol from peripheral tissues, such as the arterial wall, to the liver. Another important mechanism could be by protecting LDL against atherogenic oxidative modification, because the enzyme paraoxonase, located on HDL, can break down lipid peroxides formed on LDL and cell membranes.

Key points – lipids and lipoproteins – structure and physiology

- Low-density lipoprotein (LDL) particles are the smallest and by far the most numerous of the atherogenic particles. This explains why statin-induced LDL lowering has been so successful in reducing coronary events.
- As LDL particles differ in the amount of cholesterol they contain, LDL cholesterol level is often not an accurate guide to LDL particle number.
- The major effect of triglycerides on risk of coronary heart disease is probably from the production of small, dense LDL particles.
- High-density lipoprotein particles transport cholesterol from the periphery to the liver, though whether this is their only, or even their most important, anti-atherogenic effect is not clear.

Key references

Cahill GF. Starvation in man. *N Engl J Med* 1970;282:668–75.

Durrington PN. Lipoproteins and their metabolism. In: *Hyperlipidaemia: Diagnosis and Management*, 3rd edn. London: Hodder Arnold, 2007:19–65.

Gibbons GF, Mitropoulos K, Myant NB. *Biochemistry of Cholesterol*, 4th edn. Amsterdam: Elsevier, 1982.

Gurr MI, Harwood JL, Frayn KN. *Lipid Biochemistry: An Introduction*, 5th edn. Oxford: Blackwell Science, 2002.

Hegele RA. Monogenic dyslipidemias: window on determinants of plasma lipoprotein metabolism. *Am J Hum Genet* 2001;69:1161–77.

Packard CJ, Shepherd J. Physiology of the lipoprotein transport system: an overview of lipoprotein metabolism. In: Betteridge DJ, Illingworth DR, Shepherd J, eds. *Lipoproteins in Health and Disease*. London: Arnold, 1999:17–30.

Lipids, lipoproteins and the risk of coronary disease

Cholesterol, triglyceride and HDL cholesterol. The well-known and well-established curvilinear relationship between the level of cholesterol and the risk of coronary disease is illustrated in Figure 2.1. Over the whole range, there is a substantial increase in mortality (Figure 2.1a). However, there is no threshold below which cholesterol ceases to be a risk factor. The typical patient who develops coronary heart disease (CHD) will do so with a level of cholesterol only slightly above the average (50th percentile). However, as you can see from Figure 2.1b, if you live in the USA, even being at the 30th percentile for cholesterol is no cause for celebration because your chance of dying of CHD, although half that of someone at the 90th percentile, is still uncomfortably high. Thus, although individuals with very high levels of total and/or low-density lipoprotein (LDL) cholesterol are at substantially increased risk, unless you come from a society where typical total or LDL cholesterol levels are very low, your coronary risk is going to be unacceptably high over a wide range of cholesterol levels. Consequently, looking for particularly high cholesterol or LDL cholesterol is not a very effective way of discovering the majority of people destined to die from CHD.

Low high-density lipoprotein (HDL) cholesterol (or apoAI) is more common than high cholesterol in coronary patients. The level of HDL, whether measured as HDL cholesterol or apoAI, is accepted as a major risk factor for coronary disease. Similarly, hypertriglyceridemia is much more common in coronary patients than hypercholesterolemia (usually in combination with low HDL cholesterol).

Controversy about whether triglycerides are really a risk factor for coronary disease has raged until recently. People in the upper third of the triglyceride distribution have about 1.7 times the CHD risk of those in the lower third and this is independent of HDL levels, with which triglycerides correlate inversely. Although the risk posed by triglycerides is independent of HDL, the low HDL that frequently coexists is also likely to compound the risk in a particular individual. Other risk factors

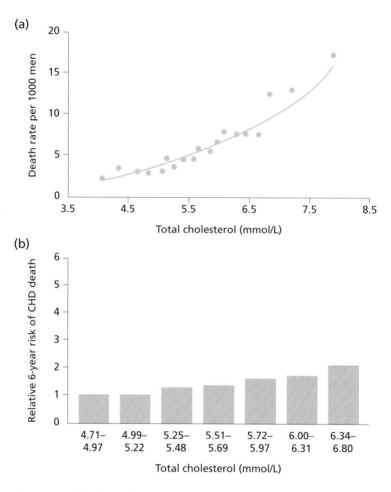

Figure 2.1 (a) Relationship between serum cholesterol levels and coronary heart disease (CHD) mortality in men. Data are from the US Multiple Risk Factor Intervention Trial (MRFIT) (LaRosa JC et al. *Circulation* 1990;81:1721–33). (b) Relative 6-year risk of CHD mortality in MRFIT from the 30th to the 90th percentile total cholesterol (Stamler J et al. *JAMA* 1986;256:2823–8).

frequently cluster with hypertriglyceridemia and this clustering is recognized by the concept of the metabolic syndrome (see Chapter 7).

Triglycerides are unlikely to contribute directly to atherosclerosis, occurring as they do in chylomicron and very-low-density lipoprotein

(VLDL) particles that are too large to cross most vascular endothelia. Evidence points strongly to the smaller chylomicron remnants and intermediate-density lipoproteins (IDL) derived from these as being the real culprits. Furthermore, high levels of triglyceride-rich lipoproteins increase the activity of cholesteryl ester transfer protein (see Chapter 1), leading to the formation of small, dense LDL particles, which are highly atherogenic. LDL cholesterol is an unreliable index of the concentration of LDL in this circumstance and that is why apoB should be measured if the test is available.

ApoB and small, dense LDL. The Apolipoprotein-related Mortality Risk Study (AMORIS) was specifically designed to compare cholesterol and apoB as markers of the risk of death from myocardial infarction in 175 553 Swedes over a 6-year follow-up period. ApoB was superior to total or LDL cholesterol in every direct comparison. ApoB was predictive above and below the age of 70 years, whereas LDL cholesterol was predictive only below the age of 70. ApoB was predictive in men and women, whereas LDL cholesterol was predictive only in men. At all levels, apoB added information about risk, though this was particularly pronounced in individuals with LDL cholesterol below the median values: < 3.73 mmol/L (150 mg/dL) in men and < 3.55 mmol/L (140 mg/dL) in women.

These are important results because they demonstrate that LDL particle number (i.e. the concentration of apoB) is a more powerful index of CHD risk than total or LDL cholesterol level. Just as important, when the findings of AMORIS are taken together with the findings of the Quebec Cardiovascular Study, they point to a better method of identifying those at high risk than is commonly followed at the moment.

Two of the most important results of the Quebec Cardiovascular Study are illustrated in Figure 2.2. When apoB is increased (i.e. when the LDL particle number is increased), but cholesterol-replete, normal-size LDL particles are present, the risk is increased twofold. By contrast, when apoB is increased and small, dense LDL particles are present, the risk is increased sixfold. Thus, increased numbers of small, dense LDL particles are particularly dangerous. Because small, dense LDL particles are depleted in cholesterol, accurate diagnosis cannot be made by

21

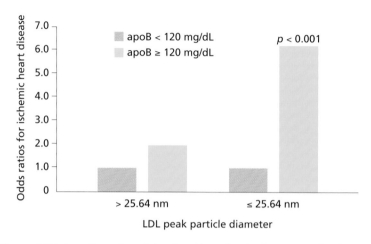

Figure 2.2 Interaction of apoB level and low-density lipoprotein (LDL) particle size as determinants of coronary heart disease risk. (Lamarche B et al. *Circulation* 1997;95:69.)

measuring serum LDL cholesterol: serum apoB measurement is necessary. Increased numbers of small, dense LDL particles are most likely to be present when triglycerides are raised and HDL is low.

ApoAI. Mounting evidence suggests that measuring the protein components of HDL, particularly apoAI, gives a better indication of risk than HDL cholesterol. Certainly in the INTERHEART study (involving 52 countries, with 15 512 cases and 14 820 controls), the ratio of apoB to apoAI was the single most important risk factor, accounting for just over 50% of myocardial infarctions (Figure 2.3).

LDL as the final common pathway to atherosclerosis

The frequency with which atherogenic lipoprotein particles encounter and enter the arterial wall is determined by their number and their size. LDL particles are more atherogenic than VLDL particles because the former are nine times more numerous and are smaller. On both these grounds, LDL qualifies as the most dangerous of the atherogenic lipoproteins.

It is useful to think of LDL as the final common pathway to induce atherosclerosis. This can occur in several ways. Some patients have marked hypercholesterolemia and thus a markedly increased LDL

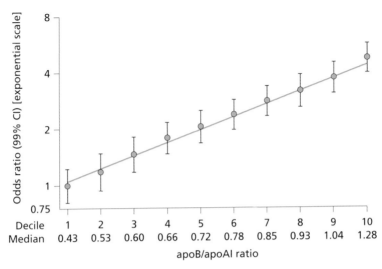

Figure 2.3 The odds of myocardial infarction related to the apoB/apoAI ratio. Adapted, with permission from Elsevier, from Yusuf S et al. 2004.

particle number, which alone may be sufficient over time to induce arterial disease. An example of this would be familial hypercholesterolemia (see Chapter 3).

But the majority of patients destined to develop atherosclerosis do not fall into this group. Most have a moderately elevated LDL particle number, or even a level that is normal for affluent Western societies. Hypertension, diabetes and smoking are generally thought to be independent risk factors for disease. Although this may be true statistically, it does not necessarily reflect the biological picture: these other risk factors modify the impact of LDL on the arterial wall. For example, hypertension increases the likelihood that an LDL particle will be forced into the vessel wall. The vessel wall is also thickened, so that an LDL particle which gets embedded in it is less likely to get out and consequently is more likely to be harmful.

As we shall see, atherogenic dyslipoproteinemias are extremely common in type 2 diabetes; but in diabetes there are additional pathogenic factors at work. Glycation of the glycosaminoglycans of the vessel wall and the lipoprotein particles themselves increases the likelihood of an LDL particle sticking within the vessel wall and then being oxidized and promoting atherogenesis. The albuminuria common in diabetes may be one facet of a more generalized leakiness of blood vessels. The potential for oxidation is increased and antioxidant defenses are frequently diminished in diabetes. Similarly, smoking provides a source of oxygen free radicals and carbon monoxide, which increase the permeability of the endothelial surface to LDL particles.

Age is actually the most powerful risk factor for vascular disease and it fits nicely into this scheme as well. The risk of disease is proportional not only to the number of LDL particles in plasma and inversely to their size, but also to the duration of exposure. The longer a vessel wall is exposed, the more injurious events there will be.

We place this great emphasis on LDL because evidence indicates that LDL is the central risk factor for coronary disease. Where populations do not consume the energetically excessive, fat-rich Western diet, the incidence of vascular disease is extremely low despite high rates of smoking and hypertension; this is because LDL levels are low. Nevertheless, even in these societies, a relationship to LDL can still be traced. The second reason is the mass of evidence now available from multiple clinical trials that unequivocally demonstrates that, at virtually all levels of LDL cholesterol, lowering LDL by pharmacological therapy significantly lowers the mortality and morbidity from coronary artery disease.

Events in the arterial wall

The great Russian experimental pathologist Anitschov wrote in 1913 that 'there can be no atheroma without cholesterol'. Just as the epidemiological evidence points firmly in that direction, so does our recent understanding of the pathological processes that lead to coronary atherogenesis, and subsequent thrombosis and occlusion. Disturbingly, in parts of the world with high CHD rates, the early lesions that give rise to later atheroma are prevalent among children. These early lesions are the fatty streaks that are commonly present in the aortas of children unfortunate enough to succumb to some unrelated sudden death, such as an accident.

Fatty streaks consist of collections of cells loaded with cytoplasmic droplets of cholesterol beneath the intimal surface of an artery (Figure 2.4). These cells are called foam cells and are usually

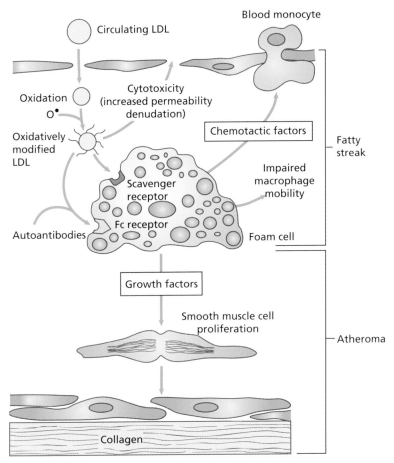

Figure 2.4 Atherogenesis: the fatty streak is characterized by lipid-laden macrophages (foam cells derived from blood monocytes attracted to the arterial subintima, where they engulf lipoproteins, such as oxidatively modified low-density lipoprotein [LDL]). Conversion of the fatty streak to atheroma depends on the proliferation and differentiation of smooth-muscle cells into fibroblasts, the elaboration of collagen and repetition of the whole process. As the lesion progresses, necrosis of foam cells leaves behind extracellular lipid deposits and an overlying fibrous cap develops (see Figure 2.6). The actively growing point of the lesion where new foam cells are forming is in the shoulder at the junction between the atheromatous lesion and the normal arterial wall. Fc, region of heavy chain of an immunoglobulin class recognized by receptors; O•, oxygen free radical.

macrophages that have internalized LDL from the tissue fluid in such quantities as to load their cytoplasm with cholesterol droplets. The initiating event in fatty streak formation is the passage of increased quantities of LDL across the endothelium of an artery into its wall. This is likely to occur at sites of turbulence, where there may be relative anoxia, when LDL levels are high and when the endothelium is damaged by, for example, hypertension, oxidation or glycation. Monocytes from the blood circulation are attracted to these sites by the damaged endothelium and themselves cross the endothelium to enter the subintimal space, where they take up LDL and assume the morphology of macrophages. Healthy, unmodified LDL is taken up only slowly, if at all, by macrophages. It must undergo some modification before it can excite foam cell formation. The modification that has attracted most recent interest has been oxidation.

Oxidation. Oxygen is two electrons short of having the same electron shell as inert neon. It forms stable compounds by sharing electrons from the outer shells of the atoms with which it reacts – for example, one from each of two hydrogen atoms to form water. Reactions of oxygen, including those catalyzed by enzymes, involve the production of an intermediate in which oxygen has acquired one additional electron in its outer shell, but has yet to receive the second to complete the reaction. At this stage, it is known as an oxygen free radical and it is highly reactive, with its outer electron shell resembling that of fluorine. Oxygen free radicals are particularly reactive at the site of double carbon bonds in organic compounds. LDL has an abundance of these in the fatty acids of the phospholipids present in its outer envelope. Oxygen free-radical attack on these phospholipids leads to the formation of lipid peroxidation products. These react with, and damage, the apoB of LDL, altering its receptor-binding characteristics. This oxidatively modified LDL is rapidly taken up by macrophages through scavenger receptors (SR-AI, SR-AII, CD36) to form foam cells.

Oxygen free radicals:
- are present in cigarette smoke
- are formed during glycation reactions

- are generated deliberately by macrophages (e.g. to kill bacteria)
- may leak from oxidative pathways.

Antioxidant mechanisms. LDL has its own fat-soluble antioxidants, which are dissolved in its central lipid droplet. They include ubiquinone, vitamin E (α- and β-tocopherol) and β-carotene.

These are chain-breaking antioxidants; they themselves react more readily with oxygen free radicals than do phospholipids. Despite the widescale consumption of vitamin E and β-carotene in the belief that they will protect against atheroma, clinical trial evidence of such an effect is unconvincing. This is perhaps because when fat-soluble antioxidants are themselves oxidized, they offer no further protection against oxidation and may even behave as pro-oxidants.

HDL appears to protect LDL against oxidative modification. It does so not by interfering with the formation of lipid peroxides on LDL, but by metabolizing them before they undergo spontaneous breakdown to form apoB-damaging substances. No pharmacological means of enhancing this activity, which is largely caused by the enzyme paraoxonase located on HDL, is yet known, but a healthy diet may help. The best policy for decreasing the production of oxidatively modified LDL is to reduce the quantity of LDL in the circulation.

Effects of oxidatively modified LDL. These are not confined to foam cell formation. Oxidatively modified LDL can also directly damage endothelial cells, stimulate the formation of autoantibodies, and excite macrophages and endothelial cells to secrete chemotactic factors that attract circulating monocytes. Foam cells themselves can produce growth factors that recruit smooth muscle cells located further out in the aortic wall into the fatty streak region. These smooth muscle cells differentiate into fibroblasts and lay down collagen. This response, which is clearly part of an inappropriately activated tissue repair process, leads to the development of the atheromatous plaque, the mature atheromatous lesion (Figure 2.5).

Other atherogenic modifications of LDL. It is increasingly realised that glycation of LDL is an atherogenic modification leading to foam cell

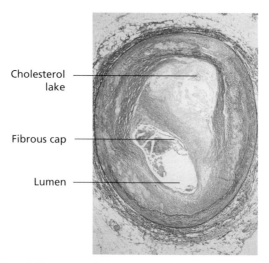

Cholesterol lake

Fibrous cap

Lumen

Figure 2.5 Mature atheromatous lesion occluding 70% of the arterial lumen. Reproduced courtesy of the Department of Pathological Sciences, Manchester Royal Infirmary, UK.

formation by a mechanism similar to that described for oxidatively modified LDL. LDL glycation occurs in the circulation of diabetic and non-diabetic people and depends largely on the concentration of small, dense LDL, which is the most susceptible lipoprotein.

Plaque formation. The collagen elaborated by fibroblasts comes to overlie the macrophage foam cells, which undergo either necrosis or apoptosis. This results in the formation of a pool of extracellular cholesterol trapped beneath a fibrous cap. The shoulder of the atheromatous lesion (where the fibrous cap joins the normal arterial wall) continues to be active, and it is here that active foam cell formation continues as the lesion advances across the inner surface of the artery (Figure 2.6). The fibrous cap is also at its most mechanically weak in this region; the secretion of collagenase from the macrophage foam cells may exacerbate this weakness. The part of the cap that ruptures is almost invariably in the shoulder of the plaque. Cholesterol-rich plaques are particularly liable to rupture their overlying fibrous cap. This becomes less likely as the quantity of fibrous tissue binding down the cap increases. Asymptomatic lesions, which occlude only 40–50% of the

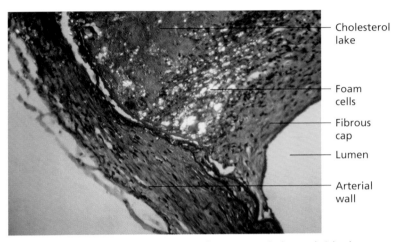

Cholesterol lake

Foam cells

Fibrous cap

Lumen

Arterial wall

Figure 2.6 The active shoulder region of a mature, cholesterol-rich plaque. The foam cells are clearly active (the orange-red material is lipid stained with Oil Red O), and pale intracellular cholesterol crystals are also present. The fibrous cap is most vulnerable to rupture here. Reproduced courtesy of the Department of Pathological Sciences, Manchester Royal Infirmary, UK.

coronary artery lumen at a stage when they are particularly rich in cholesterol, may be more liable to rupture their caps than larger, more fibrous, lesions that obstruct the artery sufficiently to cause stable angina.

Rupture of a fibrous cap may lead to discharge of the cholesterol lake from beneath it. Should healing of the broken surface then occur uneventfully, a largely fibrous atheromatous lesion will result. However, if the victim of plaque rupture is unfortunate, thrombosis will occur at the raw site of the ruptured cap (Figure 2.7). Extension of this thrombosis will cause acute occlusion of the coronary artery lumen, resulting in myocardial infarction or unstable angina.

Factors that may ultimately determine the fate of a person harboring coronary atheroma include:

- those promoting plaque rupture, such as a high circulating concentration of LDL cholesterol (contributing to formation of plaques enriched in cholesterol relative to collagen and heightening foam cell activity in the vulnerable parts of the plaque) and/or sudden rises in blood pressure
- those that make thrombosis more likely, such as cigarette smoking and diabetes, which increase circulating plasma fibrinogen levels

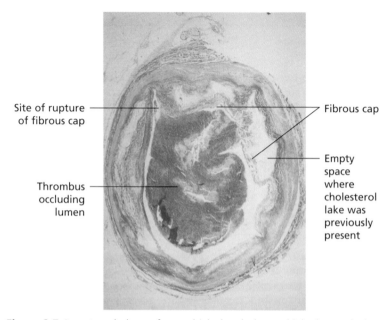

Figure 2.7 A ruptured plaque from which the cholesterol lake beneath the fibrous cap has discharged. A thrombus has formed at the raw endothelial surface of the rupture site, and the lumen is completely occluded. Reproduced courtesy of the Department of Pathological Sciences, Manchester Royal Infirmary, UK.

- the extent of myocardial damage when occlusion occurs or the propensity of the ischemic myocardium to dysrhythmia.

The scale of the problem

The UK population probably has the highest serum cholesterol levels in the world. CHD rates in the west of Scotland and Northern Ireland have recently been exceeded by those of the Czech Republic and Russia, so it is possible that other countries are in contention. Nevertheless, it is probably the worst single cause of ill health and premature death in the UK. Two-thirds of the UK population have serum cholesterol levels exceeding the optimal upper limit for a population, 5.0 mmol/L (200 mg/dL). The situation is better in the USA, where both serum cholesterol and CHD rates are lower. They are not, however, sufficiently low that there can be any grounds for complacency.

TABLE 2.1

Current working classification of hyperlipoproteinemias

- High low-density lipoprotein cholesterol with normal triglycerides: found in familial hypercholesterolemia and polygenic hypercholesterolemia

- Combined hyperlipidemia: triglycerides and low-density lipoprotein (LDL) cholesterol are elevated

- Moderate hypertriglyceridemia: triglycerides are moderately raised but LDL cholesterol is normal

- Severe hypertriglyceridemia or type V hyperlipoproteinemia: triglycerides exceed 10 mmol/L (1000 mg/dL)

- Dysbetalipoproteinemia: chylomicron remnants accumulate (remnant removal disease or type III hyperlipoproteinemia, see Chapter 6)

- Low high-density lipoprotein cholesterol with or without other abnormalities

A note on classification of hyperlipoproteinemias

The various forms of hyperlipoproteinemia used to be designated type I to type V, depending on whether chylomicron triglyceride, VLDL triglyceride or both were elevated, and whether LDL cholesterol was or was not raised as well. This convention has largely fallen into disuse, though type III and type V are terms still used in lipid clinics. The current working classification is shown in Table 2.1.

Key points – epidemiology and pathophysiology

- The atherogenic lipoproteins, particularly low-density lipoprotein, form the final common pathway to the creation of atherosclerotic lesions.
- Blood pressure, diabetes mellitus, smoking and inflammation increase the entry of atherogenic lipoproteins into the arterial wall and increase the likelihood of plaque rupture.

Key references

Barter PJ, Ballantyne CM, Carmena R et al. Apo B versus cholesterol in estimating cardiovascular risk and in guiding therapy: report of the thirty-person/ten-country panel. *J Intern Med* 2006;259:247–58.

Charlton J, Murphy M, Khaw K et al. Cardiovascular diseases. In: Charlton J, Murphy M, eds. *The Health of Adult Britain 1841–1994*, vol 2. London: TSO, 1997:60–81.

Charlton J, Quaife K. Trends in diet 1841–1994. In: Charlton J, Murphy M, eds. *The Health of Adult Britain 1841–1994*, vol 1. London: TSO, 1997:93–113.

Gordon DJ. Epidemiology of lipoproteins. In: Betteridge DJ, Illingworth DR, Shepherd J, eds. *Lipoproteins in Health and Disease*. London: Arnold, 1999:587–95.

Law MR, Wald NJ, Thompson SG. By how much and how quickly does reduction in serum cholesterol concentration lower risk of ischaemic heart disease? *BMJ* 1994;308:367–72.

Lusis AJ. Atherosclerosis. *Nature* 2000;407:233–41.

Sarwar N, Danesh J, Eiriksdottir G et al. Triglycerides and the risk of coronary heart disease: 10,158 incident cases among 262,525 participants in 29 Western prospective studies. *Circulation* 2007;115:450–8.

Sniderman AD, Furberg CD, Keech A et al. Apolipoproteins versus lipids as indices of coronary risk and as targets for statin treatment. *Lancet* 2003;361:777–80.

Steinberg D. Low density lipoprotein oxidation and its pathobiological significance. *J Biol Chem* 1997;272:20963–6.

Yusuf S, Hawken S, Ounpuu S et al. INTERHEART Study Investigators. Effect of potentially modifiable risk factors associated with myocardial infarction in 52 countries (the INTERHEART study): case–control study. *Lancet* 2004;364:937–52.

Heterozygous familial hypercholesterolemia

Genetic basis. Familial hypercholesterolemia (FH) is the most common genetic disorder in Europe and the USA, affecting about 1 in 500 people in its heterozygous form. It is not the most common cause of hypercholesterolemia. Polygenic hypercholesterolemia and combined hyperlipidemia are more common (see Chapter 4). FH is dominantly inherited and has been recognized clinically for 80 years. Its genetic basis was revealed in 1974 when Goldstein and Brown discovered the low-density lipoprotein (LDL) receptor and found its expression to be diminished in fibroblasts from patients with FH. It is now known that the gene for the LDL receptor is located on chromosome 19.

The LDL receptor allows LDL in the tissue fluid to be taken up by cells. Newly synthesized receptors migrate to the cell surface where they can bind LDL. They move through the cell membrane to the region of the cell surface containing the coated pits. At these sites, active invagination of the cell membrane occurs, which internalizes a variety of receptors and their bound ligands. The LDL receptor–LDL particle complex dissociates within a lysosome. The LDL receptors are released back into the cytoplasm and travel back to the cell membrane so that the whole cycle can be repeated. The vesicles containing LDL fuse to form larger vesicles, called endosomes, into which enzymes are secreted that break down the apoB and esterified cholesterol to amino acids and free cholesterol, respectively. The cholesterol can then enter the cytoplasm and equilibrate with the sterol in the other cell organelles.

In FH, a mutation of the receptor prevents it from participating efficiently in LDL uptake because it cannot be transported to the cell surface, it cannot bind properly to LDL once it gets there, it cannot be internalized, or it is not released from the endosome. In FH heterozygotes, one of the LDL-receptor genes has a mutation; in homozygous FH, both do. Well before the discovery of the LDL-receptor defect, it was shown that the time LDL spent in the circulation before its removal was

33

increased from the normal 2.5 days to about 4.5 days in FH heterozygotes and even longer in FH homozygotes (Figure 3.1). Impaired LDL uptake is the explanation for this observation.

In large societies in which the overall frequency of FH is low, such as the UK and the USA, more than 1000 LDL receptor mutations have been found to cause the clinical syndrome of FH. By contrast, in other societies FH is caused by a small number of mutations, and the frequency may exceed 1 in 500. These societies tend to be ones that have arisen relatively recently from a small number of early settlers or migrants – for example, in South Africa, two of the three common mutations can be traced back to two of the early Dutch settlers and the other to a Huguenot migrant. A similar situation appears to exist among descendants of French Canadian settlers within a relatively remote region of Quebec. It has been suggested that a Crusader introduced the LDL-receptor mutation that now accounts for the high prevalence of FH in Lebanon.

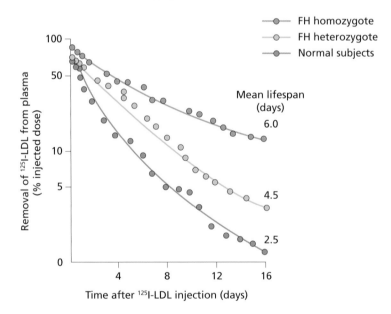

Figure 3.1 Radiolabeled low-density lipoprotein (LDL) disappears from the circulation more slowly in patients with familial hypercholesterolemia (FH) than in normal controls. Data from Bilheimer DW et al. *J Clin Invest* 1979;64:524–33.

In families with members affected by FH, marriage to close relatives for cultural or religious reasons is also likely to increase greatly the likelihood of producing a family member with homozygous FH.

Cholesterol measurements. Serum cholesterol in heterozygous FH is raised from birth – normal mean serum cholesterol concentration in umbilical cord blood is only 1.7–2.0 mmol/L (68–80 mg/dL). However, screening using total serum cholesterol is not recommended at this stage because high high-density lipoprotein (HDL) cholesterol (the dominant lipoprotein in fetal blood) is much more common than FH as a cause of high cord-blood cholesterol levels. Serum cholesterol rises in the first year of life to a mean of 4.0 mmol/L (160 mg/dL; 95th percentile, 5.0 mmol/L or 200 mg/dL) and persists until the early teens, with mean levels being similar in boys and girls before puberty. The normal range for serum cholesterol varies little with age during childhood; this allows a diagnostic threshold for childhood FH to be defined and explains why a total serum cholesterol above 6.5 mmol/L (260 mg/dL) identifies 95% of heterozygotes and only 2.5% of unaffected children. It is, of course, important to confine cholesterol measurements to the children of affected parents, so that the chances of the condition occurring are one in two. If children in general were screened, the chance of finding a heterozygote would be 1 in 500, so even a 2.5% false-positive rate would falsely identify ten unaffected children for every one affected. If the serum cholesterol exceeds 7.0 mmol/L (280 mg/dL) in childhood, FH has, almost invariably, been inherited. In families with FH, measuring cholesterol in childhood can lead to uncertainty if serum cholesterol is 5.5–7.0 mmol/L (220–280 mg/dL), particularly if the family has already adopted a cholesterol-lowering diet or the young person is experiencing the pubertal growth spurt. The diagnosis cannot then be made or excluded with complete confidence, and measurements should be repeated over time or, as DNA-based methods become increasingly available, a DNA-based diagnosis should be sought. This is much easier and cheaper, of course, if the mutation present in another family member has already been identified.

With advancing age, the serum cholesterol in FH, as in the general population, increases. In heterozygous FH, it is generally double what it would have been in the absence of the LDL-receptor mutation. For example, in a young adult woman whose serum cholesterol might have been only 4.0 mmol/L (160 mg/dL) had she not inherited the disorder, a level of 8.0 mmol/L (320 mg/dL) may indicate FH. By adulthood, the serum cholesterol in heterozygous FH is, however, typically in the range 9.0–14.0 mmol/L (360–560 mg/dL).

Tendon xanthomata, corneal arcus and xanthelasmata. Tendon xanthomata are the diagnostic hallmarks of FH. The only other causes of these, cerebrotendinous xanthomata and phytosterolemia, are so rare that for practical purposes, in the presence of tendon xanthomata, the diagnosis of FH is never really in doubt. Xanthomata are localized infiltrates of lipid-containing foam cells that histologically resemble atheroma.

Corneal arcus (Figure 3.2) and xanthelasmata (Figure 3.3) are not specific for FH, though they often occur much earlier in life in people with FH than in those with the more common polygenic type of hypercholesterolemia (see Chapter 4). Corneal arcus, for example, in the late teens or twenties may well indicate FH. On the other hand, xanthelasmata not infrequently occur in women during their first pregnancy when their serum cholesterol increases from a level that is not normally particularly high. A great many FH heterozygotes with obvious tendon xanthomata do not have corneal arcus until much later, however, and will never develop xanthelasmata. Tendon xanthomata

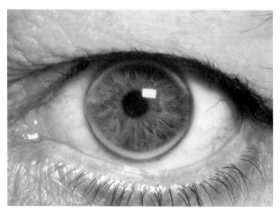

Figure 3.2
Corneal arcus.

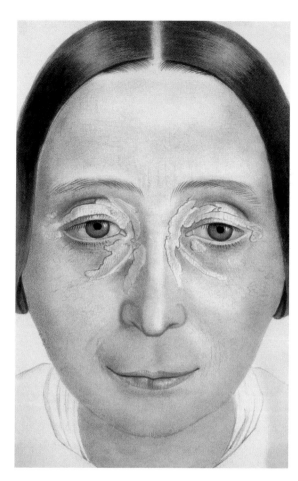

Figure 3.3 Eliza Parachute, the first patient described with xanthelasmata (Addison and Gull, Guy's Hospital Reports 1851;series II, 7:265–70).

should, therefore, be sought in all patients with hypercholesterolemia, regardless of the presence of corneal arcus or xanthelasmata.

The most common sites for tendon xanthomata are in the tendons overlying the knuckles and in the Achilles tendons (Figure 3.4). Less commonly, they may be found in the extensor hallucis longus and triceps tendons, and occasionally they occur in others. It is quite common to find xanthomata on the tibial tuberosity at the site of insertion of the patellar tendon (Figure 3.5). These are called subperiosteal xanthomata and are firmly attached to the bone.

It must be emphasized that the skin overlying tendon xanthomata and subperiosteal xanthomata has a normal color and does not appear

37

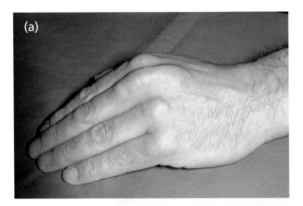

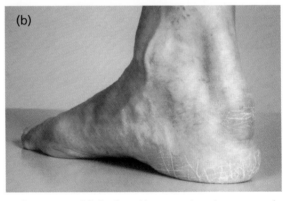

Figure 3.4 Tendon xanthomata on (a) the knuckle, reproduced courtesy of Dr JH Barth, Leeds General Infirmary, UK, and (b) the Achilles tendon.

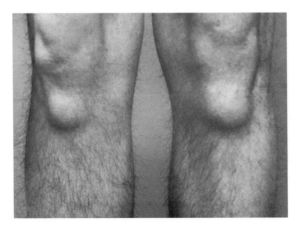

Figure 3.5
Subperiosteal xanthomata over tibial tuberosities.

yellow. The cholesterol accumulation is deep within the tendons, and much of the mass is fibrous. That is why xanthomata feel hard. Those in the Achilles tendons have a tendency to become inflamed, and many patients with FH will, if asked, give a history of earlier episodes of Achilles tenosynovitis. Xanthomata in the tendons on the dorsum of the hands are generally nodular or fusiform and, because they often overlie the knuckles (particularly when the fist is clenched) and are as hard as bone, physicians may miss them. The hand should be examined with the fingers extended – the xanthomata move back and can be moved from side to side. Achilles tendon xanthomata may be obvious, if sought, because of thickening, swelling, irregularity or nodularity of the tendon on visual inspection. They may, however, be more subtle, with the nodularity on the tendon becoming obvious only on palpation.

Family history. The other striking feature of FH is often the adverse family history of coronary heart disease (CHD), though in societies such as those of northern Europe and North America, a family history of early-onset CHD is common in the general population. Nonetheless, because FH is treatable, its diagnosis should always be sought when such a history is encountered. It is hypercholesterolemia that is inherited in FH, not necessarily the propensity to premature CHD. In some families, FH seems particularly devastating, causing CHD in men in their twenties and women before the menopause. In others, men are unaffected until late middle age and occasionally older, and women may survive to extreme old age with minimal CHD symptoms.

The general level of CHD risk can be appreciated from Table 3.1. The median age for the development of CHD in men is around 50 years. Typically, affected women in the same family develop CHD about 9 years later than their male relatives with FH. Furthermore, the penetrance of FH judged in terms of CHD risk tends to 'breed true' in families. Thus, it is striking how often one encounters a family in whom all the affected male members developed CHD at a similar age and their affected female relatives some 9 years later. This can be helpful clinically – for example, when making decisions as to the age at which to introduce lipid-lowering medication. If the family history is particularly

TABLE 3.1

Coronary heart disease (CHD) incidence and mortality associated with untreated heterozygous familial hypercholesterolemia*

Age (years)	CHD incidence (%)		CHD mortality (%)	
	Men	Women	Men	Women
< 30	5	0	0	0
30–39	22	2	7	0
40–49	48	7	25	1
50–59	80	51	52	15
60–69	100	75	78	23

*Compilation of studies in the UK (Slack J. *Lancet* 1969;2:1380–2), the USA (Stone NJ et al. *Circulation* 1974;49:476–88) and France (Beaumont V et al. *Atherosclerosis* 1976;24:441–50).

adverse, this might be in early adolescence in male heterozygotes. In other families in which the hypercholesterolemia is pursuing a more benign course, medication may be started later; for example, for women from such families, the introduction of cholesterol-lowering medication can be left until they are in their thirties, if they wish.

Tenosynovitis. In addition to Achilles tendonitis, a more generalized tenosynovitis may occur in FH. This is most commonly seen when cholesterol is lowered abruptly by, for example, partial ileal bypass, but it can also occur when cholesterol is lowered with other therapies, such as statins, when it may be wrongly attributed to the drug itself. It is due to the mobilization of cholesterol widely deposited in the tendons and periarticular tissues, and is akin to the exacerbations of gout that may accompany the mobilization of uric acid when allopurinol is introduced for the first time.

Homozygous FH

This is rare when it occurs by chance. The odds of two unrelated heterozygotes marrying is 1 in 250 000 (unless, of course, they meet at a lipid clinic) and the chances of them having a child who is homozygous is 1 in 4, making the theoretical incidence of homozygous FH one in a million. The chances of a marriage between heterozygotes are greatly increased when there is, for example, a tradition of first-cousin marriage. In such circumstances, both of the LDL-receptor mutations in homozygotes are likely to be the same, and the affected person is a true homozygote. Homozygotes arising from random union are likely to have a different LDL-receptor mutation on each chromosome and are, in reality, compound heterozygotes (though they are classified as homozygotes).

Homozygous FH is always a serious problem. Serum cholesterol levels are almost invariably greater than 15 mmol/L (600 mg/dL) and can be as high as 30 mmol/L (1200 mg/dL). Most homozygotes develop angina of effort in childhood resulting from the aortic stenosis and coronary atheroma. Myocardial infarction has been recorded as early as at 2 years, and life expectancy does not usually extend beyond the early twenties. The very worst prognosis seems to occur when both LDL-receptor mutations are of the type that completely prevents LDL receptors appearing on the cell surface.

Signs. Xanthomata develop in childhood. In addition to florid tendon xanthomata of the type already described, orange-yellow cutaneous planar xanthomata develop, particularly in the popliteal and antecubital fossae (Figure 3.6), buttocks and in the webs between the fingers. They may develop on the palms of the hands and the fronts of the knees during crawling. Polyarthralgia is common and supravalvar aortic stenosis can cause sudden death.

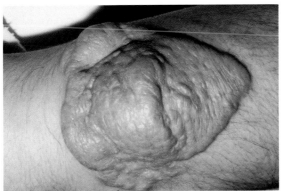

Figure 3.6
Subcutaneous planar xanthoma in the antecubital fossa. Reproduced courtesy of Dr JP Miller, University Hospital of South Manchester, UK.

FH arising from mutations in genes other than the LDL-receptor gene

Currently, 50–80% of patients in the UK and USA with a clinical diagnosis of heterozygous FH have identifiable mutations of the LDL receptor. As for the remainder, it is possible that genetic techniques are failing to detect LDL-receptor mutations or that the clinicians' diagnosis of FH is incorrect. It is also possible that there are other genes encoding proteins involved in LDL catabolism that have undergone mutation in some patients. Three of these are the gene encoding apoB (familial defective apoB), the gene encoding proprotein convertase subtilisin/kexin type 9 (PCSK9) and the autosomal recessive hypercholesterolemia (*ARH*) gene.

Familial defective apoB. Occasionally, a heterozygous FH syndrome arises because the gene encoding apoB has a mutation. The protein's ability to bind to the LDL receptor is affected, which results in a defect in LDL catabolism. This is called familial defective apoB (FDB). It most commonly results from an amino-acid substitution at position 3500. This mutation has a frequency of about 1 in 600 in the general population, though it does not generally produce a particularly severe hyperlipidemia. It has, however, been estimated that around 2–3% of people with clinical FH have FDB. Their hypercholesterolemia appears to respond more easily to treatment than is generally the case in FH.

PCSK9. A few patients with heterozygous FH have been reported in whom the gene encoding PCSK9 has undergone a 'gain of function' mutation. PCSK9 is involved in LDL-receptor degradation, which is increased in patients with this mutation, creating a defect in LDL catabolism. The resulting syndrome resembles severe heterozygous FH. Other people have been detected in whom genetic mutations lead to impaired PCSK9 function, increasing LDL catabolism, and resulting in low LDL cholesterol levels and a reduced risk of CHD.

ARH has been described largely in people of Sardinian extraction. The clinical phenotype is intermediate between homozygous and heterozygous FH. It involves a defect in LDL catabolism that is not mediated through a mutation of the LDL-receptor gene, but through the *ARH* gene, which encodes a protein involved in the internalization of receptor-bound LDL from the cell surface.

Diagnosis

FH can be diagnosed with ease if features of the clinical syndrome are present in people with hypercholesterolemia or the raised cholesterol is discovered in childhood, when other causes of hypercholesterolemia are even rarer. Unfortunately, the variety of mutations encountered in unrelated patients with FH means that no simple, widely applicable means of genetic testing is feasible, except perhaps in a country such as South Africa where a much smaller number of mutations exist. In most countries, even testing for the more common mutation will still leave more than half of patients with unidentified mutations. Thus, increasing attention is being paid to combining mutation identification with cholesterol testing in a process known as 'cascade family screening'. A person with definite features of heterozygous FH who attends a lipid clinic is diagnosed, for example using the Simon Broome criteria (Table 3.2) (this person is the 'proband', the family member through whom the family's medical history comes to light). A detailed family history, including contact details of all their first-degree relatives,

---

TABLE 3.2

Simon Broome criteria for the diagnosis of definite heterozygous familial hypercholesterolemia*

- Children under 16: total serum cholesterol ≥ 6.7 mmol/L (260 mg/dL)

- Adults: total serum cholesterol ≥ 7.5 mmol/L (290 mg/dL) or LDL cholesterol ≥ 4.9 mmol/L (190 mg/dL)

plus

- Tendon xanthomata in patient or in first- or second-degree relative

*From Neil HAW et al. *Atherosclerosis* 2005;179:293–7. For reviews of other more detailed clinical criteria, see Austin MA et al. *Am J Epidemiol* 2004;160:421–9, and Hadfield SG et al. *Curr Opin Lipidol* 2005;16:428–33.

is obtained and the relatives are traced and tested for raised cholesterol; if the mutation has been identified in the proband, a DNA test is also offered. This approach identifies new cases of FH through their clearly raised cholesterol and/or mutation. The process of tracing relatives is then repeated with them. Studies show that this approach gives a high yield of younger patients who have not yet developed coronary disease.

Ideally, FH should be diagnosed before the clinical phenotype – which includes premature CHD – has fully developed, because the aim of treatment should be to prevent or delay this complication. Late adolescence or young adulthood is not the best time to diagnose heterozygous FH; the adolescent growth spurt means the LDL cholesterol may not be as high as in childhood – this is unfortunate as it would be the most advantageous time to begin statin treatment. Furthermore, polygenic hypercholesterolemia (see Chapter 4) begins to manifest itself at this time and can confuse matters; tendon xanthomata, which would clearly identify FH, may not be present for some years to come.

It is important to emphasize that the introduction of lipid-lowering therapy is not the only reason for identifying heterozygotes for FH. The disorder is still not widely recognized. When FH patients present with manifestations of CHD, they are often inappropriately managed if seen by physicians unfamiliar with the condition. There is a general disbelief that apparently fit, young people can have severe CHD. This usually leads to a delay in investigations, particularly coronary angiography. Certainly, exercise electrocardiography should be carried out promptly when symptoms that are in the least suggestive of CHD occur, and FH patients should be encouraged to report such symptoms. Coronary angiograms often reveal surprisingly extensive disease despite relatively minimal symptoms, and should not be withheld. The pressure gradient across the aortic valve should be measured using echocardiography when a systolic murmur is present.

Management

Heterozygous FH. The statin drugs represent a major advance in the management of FH. Most people with heterozygous FH can now achieve serum cholesterol levels below 7.0 mmol/L (280 mg/dL) and some even below 5.0 mmol/L (200 mg/dL). The most potent of the statins may be required at maximum doses in patients with the higher cholesterol levels. The therapeutic response is often inadequate if judged by the targets of statin treatment for patients in general. Bile-acid-sequestrating agents or nicotinic acid can further augment the statin response. However, both are poorly tolerated, particularly at higher doses. Ezetimibe is generally well tolerated and produces an additional LDL cholesterol reduction of 15–20%. Partial ileal bypass is often successful in decreasing serum cholesterol, but it has been used less often since the advent of statins.

Homozygous FH. The cholesterol-lowering effect achieved with medication in homozygous FH is generally disappointing. Even with the most potent statins a decrease in LDL cholesterol of more than 30% is seldom achieved. Ezetimibe can achieve an additional decrease, but even then substantial hypercholesterolemia remains. Plasmapheresis or LDL apheresis is the best approach to correcting this. Generally, the procedure must be carried out every 2 weeks. Liver transplantation has also met with some success. This introduces normal donor hepatic LDL receptors. The LDL-receptor gene can be expressed in transfected LDL-receptor-knockout mice, lowering serum cholesterol, albeit only briefly before it is cleared from the cell nuclei along with viral DNA. It is hoped that homozygous FH will be one of the first genetic disorders to be treated by this technique, as soon as a vector that allows foreign DNA to persist in mammalian cells becomes available.

Genetic counseling

There is no need to suggest that a patient with heterozygous FH should limit their family as long as their partner is not also a heterozygote. It is advisable to check the partner's serum cholesterol to establish this. Although there is a 50% chance that each child of a heterozygote for FH with a non-FH partner will themselves be FH heterozygotes, the prospect for improved treatment is great and the condition not generally so severe as to suggest that such individuals will not enjoy quality of life. However, depending on the family history, it may be sensible that FH patients do not wait until the bloom of youth is too far behind them before starting their families, because of the devastating effect the death of a parent can have on young children.

CHD susceptibility

CHD is far and away the most common manifestation of atheroma in heterozygous FH. Atheromatous deposits may also occur in the root of the aorta and can extend into the aortic valve cusps; these occur particularly in homozygous FH, but also in as many as 30% of heterozygotes. This form of supravalvar aortic stenosis and aortic sclerosis may be the cause of an aortic systolic murmur. Some patients also develop carotid and intracerebral atheroma, though not as frequently as CHD. Femoropopliteal atheroma is also less common than CHD and is really only encountered in cigarette smokers with FH.

There has been much speculation as to why some families with FH are more susceptible to CHD than others. The nature of the mutation may itself be important, because some mutations compromise LDL uptake more severely than others. The particular combination of mutations certainly influences the severity of homozygous FH, but this is less clear in heterozygous FH. Indeed, neither the pretreatment LDL cholesterol level nor the extent and size of tendon xanthomata is clearly related to prognosis in FH.

Serum HDL cholesterol is, however, related to the likelihood of CHD in FH. Serum HDL cholesterol is generally lower than expected in FH, and prognosis is often poor in families where this is most obvious. Usually in FH, only the serum cholesterol is raised as a consequence of the increase in LDL. Triglycerides are elevated in a minority of patients, though seldom to more than 4.0 mmol/L (360 mg/dL). This, too, has been associated with a worse prognosis. These people are often obese, and obesity can increase serum cholesterol, sometimes even to 20 mmol/L (800 mg/dL) or more.

Obesity is generally uncommon in FH – in contrast to all other hyperlipidemias, in which obesity is over represented. Hypertension and diabetes mellitus are noticeably uncommon in FH; again, this is unlike other hyperlipoproteinemias. Cigarette smoking may be more common in some families with a worse prognosis, and socioeconomic deprivation almost certainly worsens the outlook. Co-inheritance of the *ApoE4* allele or of high serum lipoprotein (a) may also be associated with a worse prognosis.

Key points – familial (monogenic) hypercholesterolemia

- Heterozygous FH carries a particularly high risk of coronary heart disease and requires early treatment.
- Diagnosis is critical. Fortunately, familial hypercholesterolemia (FH) families have a distinctive clinical picture.
- Homozygous FH is much rarer but unfortunately remains a treatment challenge.

Key references

Abifadel M, Varret M, Rabes JP et al. Mutations in PCSK9 cause autosomal dominant hypercholesterolemia. *Nat Genet* 2003;34:154–6.

Arca M, Zuliani G, Wilund K et al. Autosomal recessive hypercholesterolaemia in Sardinia, Italy, and mutations in ARH: a clinical and molecular genetic analysis. *Lancet* 2002;359:841–7.

Durrington PN. Familial hypercholesterolaemia. In: *Hyperlipidaemia: Diagnosis and Management*, 3rd edn. London: Hodder Arnold, 2007:92–124.

Goldstein JL, Hobbs HH, Brown MD. Familial hyper-cholesterolaemia. In: Scriver CR, Beaudet AL, Sly WS et al., eds. *The Metabolic and Molecular Bases of Inherited Disease*, 8th edn. New York: McGraw-Hill, 2001: 2863–913.

McCrindle BW, Urbina EM, Dennison BA et al. Drug therapy of high-risk lipid abnormalities in children and adolescents: a scientific statement from the American Heart Association Atherosclerosis, Hypertension, and Obesity in Youth Committee, Council on Cardiovascular Disease in the Young, with the Council on Cardiovascular Nursing. *Circulation* 2007;115:1948–67.

National Institute for Health and Clinical Excellence. Identification and Management of Familial Hypercholesterolaemia. *Clinical Guideline* 71. London: National Institute for Health and Clinical Excellence, 2008. Available from www.nice.org.uk/guidance/CG71

Wiegman A, de Groot E, Hutten BA et al. Arterial intima-media thickness in children heterozygous for familial hypercholesterolaemia. *Lancet* 2004;363:369–70.

Polygenic hypercholesterolemia and combined hypercholesterolemia and hypertriglyceridemia (combined hyperlipidemia) are much more common than familial hypercholesterolemia (FH) as causes of elevated low-density lipoprotein (LDL) cholesterol. In Europe and North America, FH probably accounts for no more than 3% of men dying of coronary heart disease (CHD) before the age of 60.

Polygenic hypercholesterolemia

Figure 4.1a illustrates schematically a normal complement of very-low-density lipoprotein (VLDL) and LDL particles. There are nine times more LDL than VLDL particles, and most of the LDL particles are cholesterol replete. Because particle number is normal, total cholesterol, triglyceride, LDL cholesterol and apoB are all normal.

Figure 4.1b illustrates the lipoprotein profile in a patient with polygenic hypercholesterolemia. The patient either has a normal number of VLDL particles or, if their number is increased as a consequence of overproduction, the VLDL particles contain less triglyceride. Plasma triglyceride levels are not increased. However, there are increased numbers of LDL particles, which are normal in composition. Therefore, total cholesterol, LDL cholesterol and apoB are all increased.

In most instances, the increased LDL level is due to overproduction of LDL particles rather than impaired clearance. Overproduction of LDL would lead to an increased LDL particle number because the capacity of even the normal LDL pathway to remove LDL particles from plasma is limited. The level of small, dense LDL is generally not increased in these patients. The risk of coronary disease is increased, but not as markedly as in combined hyperlipidemia.

Combined hyperlipidemia

This is the commonest dyslipoproteinemia in patients with premature vascular disease. It is also among the most common dyslipoproteinemias

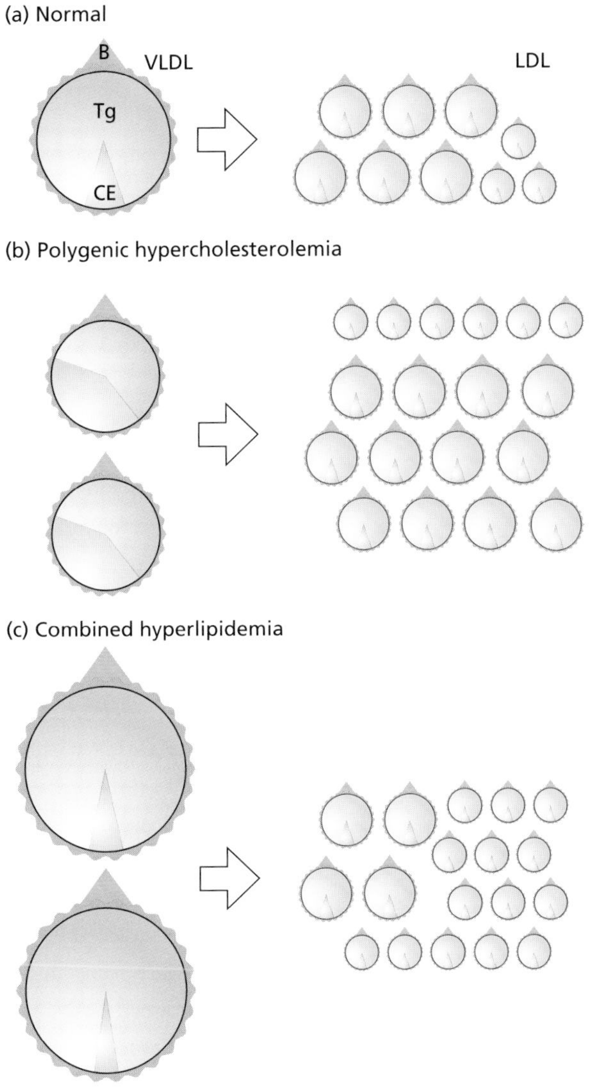

Figure 4.1 Lipoprotein profiles: (a) normal; (b) polygenic hypercholesterolemia; (c) combined hyperlipidemia. B, apolipoprotein B; CE, cholesteryl ester; LDL, low-density lipoprotein; Tg, triglyceride; VLDL, very-low-density lipoprotein.

in patients with type 2 diabetes and/or abdominal obesity. Furthermore, it is the characteristic dyslipoproteinemia of familial combined hyperlipidemia (FCHL), the commonest familial dyslipoproteinemia associated with premature coronary artery disease.

Figure 4.1c illustrates the typical lipoprotein profile in these patients. Both VLDL and LDL particle numbers are increased, producing both hypercholesterolemia and hypertriglyceridemia. VLDL production by the liver is increased and the VLDL particles are large and rich in triglyceride. This produces the ideal conditions for the generation of small, dense LDL, which are also increased in concentration. Because most LDL particles are cholesterol-depleted, the apoB and, therefore, the LDL particle numbers are even higher than would be predicted from the LDL cholesterol. Note that high-density lipoprotein cholesterol is often low in these patients, further increasing risk.

The pathophysiology of combined hyperlipidemia runs as follows. During both fasting and the postprandial period, there tends to be excessive release of fatty acids from adipose tissue, which leads to increased delivery of fatty acids to the liver. Increased delivery of fatty acids results in increased hepatic triglyceride and cholesterol synthesis, leading to an increased secretion rate of VLDL particles packed with as much triglyceride as possible.

Diabetes and insulin resistance are common in these patients, probably because of the multiple adverse effects of fatty acids on glucose and insulin metabolism. Excess fatty acids cause insulin resistance: first because they oppose insulin-induced glucose uptake by muscle, and second because they inhibit the normal insulin-mediated suppression of hepatic VLDL secretion. This puts greater demand on the pancreas to maintain higher insulin levels to overcome these effects – a demand which individuals susceptible to diabetes cannot meet.

Familial combined hyperlipidemia. Originally, FCHL was thought to be a dominantly inherited hyperlipidemia closely associated with CHD, but differing from FH in that both hypercholesterolemia and hypertriglyceridemia were running within the same family and occurring singly or in combination in individual members. That is, within an affected family there were, with roughly equal frequency, those with a combined increase in cholesterol and triglycerides, those with an increase in triglycerides only and those with an increase in cholesterol only. In the original series of studies, this disorder was at least ten times more common than FH.

Subsequent research has not supported the concept of simple dominant inheritance, though genetic factors are clearly at work in affected families. FCHL remains an important clinical syndrome even though it is less easy to define than FH. In contrast to FH, hyperlipidemia does not generally appear in subjects with FCHL until early middle age, though an elevated apoB may be present much earlier. In addition, hypertension and hyperinsulinemia and/or hyperglycemia are commonly associated with FCHL, but not with FH. FCHL, like polygenic hypercholesterolemia, but again unlike FH, has as its root cause overproduction of VLDL, even in those affected individuals whose serum triglycerides are not raised.

Diagnosis. Affected individuals may be normolipidemic, hypertriglyceridemic, hypercholesterolemic, or hypertriglyceridemic and hypercholesterolemic, but all have elevated levels of apoB and small, dense LDL.

The elevated apoB is the consequence of increased secretion of VLDL particles. Depending on the composition of the VLDL secreted by the liver, and probably more importantly on the peripheral activity of lipoprotein lipase (LPL), plasma triglycerides may be normal or elevated. They usually, however, exceed 1.5 mmol/L (130 mg/dL). Whether total and LDL cholesterol are normal or elevated depends on:

- the number of small, dense LDL particles that are present
- how cholesterol depleted they are
- the efficiency of the LDL pathway.

It must be emphasized that the prime target of therapy in these patients is to reduce the atherogenic particle number – that is, to reduce the elevated plasma apoB.

Pathogenesis. Much remains to be learned about the pathogenesis of FCHL. We think it is unlikely that a single gene will prove responsible. Rather, any of several genes, individually or collectively, that impinge on a critical metabolic process such as the effectiveness of adipose tissue at storing fatty acids are likely to be the culprits. Another cluster of genes which has often been implicated in FCHL is on chromosome 11, where the genes for apolipoproteins AI, CIII, AIV and AV lie adjacent to each other. Variants of the gene encoding LPL may also be important in some families.

Role of diet

Obesity and a high-fat diet (particularly one high in saturated fat) are probably the major reasons for the enormous variations worldwide in the prevalence of polygenic hypercholesterolemia and combined hyperlipidemia. Undoubtedly, individual responses to diet vary tremendously, and there is probably a complex interplay between dietetic and genetic factors in the genesis of the disorders.

There is an impression that dietary modification aimed at lowering cholesterol in middle age in societies in which serum cholesterol is high does not reduce it to the extent that might be expected. Whether this is simply a matter of non-compliance with diet or whether it represents some permanent change in metabolism caused by a high-fat diet in early life is uncertain.

Physical signs

Tendon xanthomata are absent in both polygenic hyper-cholesterolemia and combined hyperlipidemia. Their presence in a patient with combined hyperlipidemia highly favors a diagnosis of the unusual co-occurrence of FH and hypertriglyceridemia.

Xanthelasmata and corneal arcus occur in all types of hypercholesterolemia. In patients with both hypercholesterolemia and hypertriglyceridemia, tuberoeruptive or striate palmar xanthomata generally indicate that the patient has familial dysbetalipoproteinemia (see Chapter 6). Eruptive xanthomata are associated with severe hypertriglyceridemia with hyperchylomicronemia.

Obesity, particularly android obesity, is common in patients with combined hyperlipidemia.

Role of lipid-lowering medication

When primary hypercholesterolemia is marked or linked with hypertriglyceridemia, and there is an adverse family history of CHD, there is a strong case for introducing statin treatment. The age at which this should be done is often also determined by the family history. Unhealthy cholesterol levels are, however, prevalent in coronary-disease-prone societies, such as those of the USA and Europe. There is enormous variation between individuals in the risk posed by a particular elevation in cholesterol. Other factors must be taken into account when estimating an individual's cardiovascular risk. Otherwise lipid-lowering medication will be taken by people who stand to gain little benefit and healthcare systems will be bankrupted. How to estimate risk and the thresholds for the introduction of lipid-lowering medication are discussed in Chapter 11.

Key points – polygenic hypercholesterolemia and combined hyperlipidemia

- Polygenic hypercholesterolemia and combined hyperlipidemia are two of the most common, and therefore two of the most important, atherogenic dyslipoproteinemias.
- All other things being equal, the prognosis of combined hyperlipidemia is worse than that of polygenic hypercholesterolemia.
- Individuals with either phenotype may come from a family with familial combined hyperlipidemia.

Key references

Durrington PN. Common hyperlipidaemia: familial combined hyperlipidaemia and polygenic hypercholesterolaemia. In: *Hyperlipidaemia: Diagnosis and Management*, 3rd edn. London: Hodder Arnold, 2007:125–68.

Jarvik GP, Austin MA, Brunzell JD. Familial combined hyperlipidaemia. In: Betteridge DJ, Illingworth DR, Shepherd J, eds. *Lipoproteins in Health and Disease*. London: Arnold, 1999:693–9.

Sniderman AD, Zhang XJ, Cianflone K. Governance of the concentration of plasma LDL: a reevaluation of the LDL receptor paradigm. *Atherosclerosis* 2000;148:215–29.

Veerkamp MJ, de Graaf J, Hendriks JC et al. Nomogram to diagnose familial combined hyperlipidemia on the basis of results of a 5-year follow-up study. *Circulation* 2004;109:2980–5.

Treatment is necessary to avoid the risk of acute pancreatitis in extreme hypertriglyceridemia. The association of even modest hypertriglyceridemia with coronary heart disease (CHD) has also become clear in recent years. However, reducing CHD risk in individuals with hypertriglyceridemia remains a complex issue. This chapter examines separately patients with moderate hypertriglyceridemia, 1.7–10 mmol/L (150–900 mg/dL), and those with higher levels. There is no sharp division between these groups, however. Some people with apparently moderate fasting hypertriglyceridemia have the capacity, under certain circumstances, to develop gross hypertriglyceridemia leading to acute pancreatitis; others who habitually have serum triglyceride values above 30 mmol/L (2700 mg/dL) can live to a ripe old age without complications.

Moderate hypertriglyceridemia

The upper limit of normal values for fasting serum triglycerides was, until recently, quoted as 2.3 mmol/L (200 mg/dL), though the 95th percentiles for the UK and the US populations are closer to 3 mmol/L (270 mg/dL). With the increasing recognition that triglyceride levels predict CHD risk, a lower level of 1.7 mmol/L (150 mg/dL) has been adopted as one of the criteria for the diagnosis of metabolic syndrome (see Chapter 7). At this level, small, dense low-density lipoprotein (LDL) will regularly be present in the circulation.

A low high-density lipoprotein (HDL) cholesterol level frequently co-exists with raised triglyceride levels. The major reasons are:

- cholesteryl ester transfer protein activity is high in hypertriglyceridemia, so cholesteryl ester is rapidly transferred out of HDL to very-low-density lipoprotein (VLDL) (see Chapter 1)
- lipoprotein lipase (LPL) activity is commonly low in hypertriglyceridemia – this may be because of inherited low LPL activity or LPL activators, but it is also commonly the result of insulin resistance secondary to central obesity.

When LPL hydrolyzes the core triglyceride of chylomicrons and VLDL, it releases important components of HDL from their surface. If hypertriglyceridemia produces low HDL cholesterol, it makes no clinical sense to conclude that HDL cholesterol is important in atherogenesis and triglycerides are not, as has frequently been the case in the past.

With the wider appreciation that even LDL cholesterol levels once regarded as normal can be associated with significant CHD risk, we are less clear about which patients should be regarded as having raised triglycerides but normal LDL cholesterol. In a sense, the prevalence of pure hypertriglyceridemia has contracted and what is regarded as combined hyperlipidemia has expanded. What is important is that statin drugs have clearly been shown to decrease cardiovascular risk regardless of the LDL cholesterol and triglyceride levels. So when deciding who should receive them, the major consideration should be whether significant cardiovascular risk is present.

Epidemiological studies have provided evidence that raised triglycerides are a more accurate indicator of increased cardiovascular risk in patients without a history of symptomatic vascular disease than increased cholesterol, low HDL cholesterol, increased blood pressure or smoking history. In those who have already developed CHD, raised triglycerides are associated with a significantly worse prognosis.

When patients have high triglycerides, the LDL target of statin treatment poses great difficulties, as does the issue of whether to add an additional class of lipid-lowering drug. One problem, as we have previously discussed, is that an apparently low LDL cholesterol on statin treatment may hide a multitude of sins if the patient has retained a high level of the cholesterol-depleted, small, dense LDL. A second problem is that measurement of LDL cholesterol becomes difficult for many laboratories once the triglycerides exceed 4.5 mmol/L (400 mg/dL). To overcome this, the Third Adult Treatment Panel (ATPIII) of the National Cholesterol Education Program has recommended that non-HDL cholesterol (total cholesterol minus HDL cholesterol) be calculated in these patients and used rather than LDL cholesterol as an index of risk and the target for statin therapy. The non-HDL cholesterol thresholds are those for LDL cholesterol to which 0.75 mmol/L (30 mg/dL) is added (see Chapter 11). This is helpful, but a bit complicated for most clinicians and can sometimes be misleading. Ideally, we should know what the LDL level is by measuring it in terms of its apoB, which can be done regardless of the serum triglyceride level and which, unlike LDL cholesterol or non-HDL cholesterol, will reveal the true state of affairs about how much LDL can still be removed from the circulation by therapy. Until this becomes available generally, like so many decisions in medicine, we have to look deeper into the problem and realize that surrogate measures are necessarily imprecise, and common sense and clinical judgment must prevail when determining how to treat individual patients.

Diet. Obesity is common in all types of hypertriglyceridemia; dietary advice should be directed at weight reduction. In those who are not overweight, or who fail to lose weight, generally restricting saturated fats is more effective than restricting carbohydrate intake. Restriction of refined carbohydrate is sensible, though.

For patients to lose weight, decreases in overall fat intake may be required. In the case of severe hypertriglyceridemia, when the contribution of chylomicrons is significant, a restriction in the intake of all types of fat is essential. Under these circumstances, carbohydrate intake may have to be increased in lean patients. Many patients with hypertriglyceridemia are overtly diabetic. Others are glucose intolerant or will become so over the next few years. Weight reduction and dietary fat restriction improve glucose tolerance more effectively than carbohydrate restriction because both measures decrease insulin resistance. It is insulin resistance that is generally the cause of diabetes or glucose intolerance in hypertriglyceridemia, particularly when associated with CHD.

Statins. When serum triglycerides are only moderately elevated, up to say 5.0 mmol/L (450 mg/dL), a statin may be the best first-line treatment. Often no other treatment will be necessary because, in addition to their cholesterol-lowering effect, statins also decrease triglycerides, and there is strong evidence that they prevent CHD, generally without adverse effects (which is not known with the same degree of certainty for some other lipid-lowering drugs).

For some high-risk patients whose hypertriglyceridemia persists despite statin drugs, purified omega-3 fatty acids, fibrates and nicotinic acid can

57

be considered. Even though the triglyceride-lowering effect of statins may be inadequate to lower triglycerides under these circumstances, there is a strong case for combining statins with these drugs because of the strength of evidence that statins decrease cardiovascular risk. The reason is probably that they are effective in lowering small, dense LDL even when triglyceride levels remain high. Note that, because of the increased risk of myositis, a statin should only be combined with a fibrate or nicotinic acid in an informed patient and with careful monitoring.

Purified omega-3 fatty acids combined with a statin often decrease triglyceride levels satisfactorily. They have little cholesterol-decreasing effect, but there is evidence from three studies, GISSI-Prevenzione, GISSI-heart failure and the Japan Eicosapentaenoic acid (EPA) Lipid Intervention Study (JELIS), that they decrease cardiovascular risk. The same is not true of fish oil, for which there is little evidence of benefit and which may contain oils and various impurities best avoided. Fish oil is also poorly tolerated compared with purified omega-3 fatty acids.

Fibrates cannot be recommended either individually or in combination with a statin to reduce myocardial ischemic events. To be sure, there is some clinical trial evidence supporting the use of gemfibrozil, but the evidence base is restricted and gemfibrozil is the fibrate most strongly contraindicated in combination with statin treatment because of the risk of severe skeletal muscle injury. Indeed, gemfibrozil on its own poses such a risk. With regard to fenofibrate, now the most common agent of the class employed clinically, the clinical trial evidence is very disappointing, with failure to achieve the primary endpoint in the Fenofibrate Intervention and Event Lowering in Diabetes (FIELD) study (as a single agent) and in the Action to Control Cardiovascular Risk in Diabetes (ACCORD) trial (in combination with a statin). Fibrates can be helpful in cases of familial dysbetalipoproteinemia and in selected patients with severe hypertriglyceridemia.

Nicotinic acid is particularly effective at lowering both triglyceride and cholesterol levels. However, daily doses of several grams are generally required, and at this level nicotinic acid has many side effects (see

Chapter 10). These can be ameliorated by the use of a modified-release preparation combined with aspirin; trials with an inhibitor of the prostaglandin-mediated flushing induced by nicotinic acid are under way.

Effect of β-blockers. The indications for β-blockers should be reviewed, particularly if the hypertriglyceridemia is marked. Following the findings of the large Anglo-Scandinavian Cardiac Outcomes Trial (ASCOT), β-blockers are no longer seen as first-line treatment for hypertension. The evidence that β-blockers provide symptomatic relief for angina and are cardioprotective after myocardial infarction is unchallenged and these remain compelling indications.

Severe hypertriglyceridemia (types I and V hyperlipoproteinemia)

In any circumstance where serum triglycerides exceed 10 mmol/L (900 mg/dL), chylomicrons are the major contributors to the hyper-lipidemia, even when the patient is fasting. Chylomicrons and VLDL compete for the same clearance mechanism in the circulation (LPL). The lipoprotein phenotype is usually type V. This severe hypertriglyceridemia generally occurs when an increase in hepatic VLDL production, either familial or secondary to, for example, obesity, diabetes, alcohol abuse or estrogen administration, is associated with decreased triglyceride clearance. This again may be genetic or acquired: for example, in hypothyroidism, β-blockade or diabetes mellitus (diabetes can cause both overproduction of VLDL and decreased LPL activity).

With the clearance mechanism already overloaded with VLDL, the rise in serum triglyceride levels when chylomicrons enter the circulation following a fatty meal may be dramatic, and the chylomicrons may spend days rather than hours in the circulation. The serum takes on the appearance of milk (Figure 5.1), and triglyceride levels may exceed 100 mmol/L (9000 mg/dL). A patient who might otherwise have a fasting serum triglyceride level of 5 mmol/L (450 mg/dL) can, with the injudicious use of alcohol or the development of diabetes, achieve extraordinarily high serum triglyceride levels. Overall, the frequency of severe hypertriglyceridemia is probably no more than 1 in 1000 in adults, and lower in children.

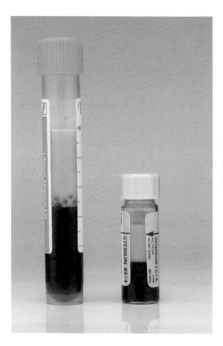

Figure 5.1 Milky serum from a patient with severe (type V) hyperlipoproteinemia.

Familial LPL deficiency. Rarely, severe hypertriglyceridemia is caused by familial LPL deficiency, a genetic deficiency in LPL activity. This is inherited as an autosomal recessive trait. It is usually caused by mutations in the gene encoding LPL, leading to defective function or production of the enzyme, but occasionally it results from a genetic deficiency of apoCII, the activator of LPL.

Severe hypertriglyceridemia may present during childhood. Occasionally in children and young adults, familial LPL deficiency produces type I hyperlipoproteinemia, in which only serum chylomicron levels are elevated. It is not known for certain why the VLDL is not also raised, but it is likely that hepatic lipase can catabolize the lower levels of VLDL produced in childhood, though it is unable to compensate for the absence of LPL as far as chylomicron catabolism is concerned. With advancing age, VLDL production increases to levels above those that can be cleared by LPL. As a result, VLDL and chylomicrons accumulate in the circulation, and type V hyperlipoproteinemia becomes apparent.

Physical signs. Eruptive xanthomata are characteristic of extreme hypertriglyceridemia. They appear as yellow papules on the extensor surfaces of the arms and legs, buttocks and back (Figure 5.2). Hepatosplenomegaly is common, and imaging shows the liver to be fatty. Bone marrow biopsy may reveal foam cells. Because the triglyceride-rich lipoprotein may interfere with the determination of transaminases, giving spuriously high values, liver disease, in particular alcoholic liver disease, may be difficult to exclude other than by the prompt resolution of the syndrome when a low-fat diet is instituted. Other features include lipemia retinalis, with both the retinal veins and arteries appearing white (Figure 5.3).

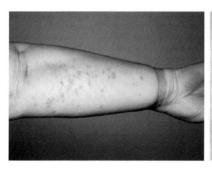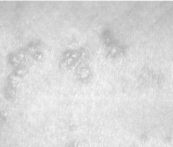

Figure 5.2 Eruptive xanthomata in a patient with severe (type V) hyperlipoproteinemia.

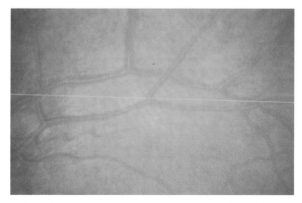

Figure 5.3 Lipemia retinalis. Reproduced courtesy of Dr JP Miller, University Hospital of South Manchester, UK.

Atheroma is not a complication of familial LPL deficiency, but it does complicate severe hypertriglyceridemia in which there is LPL activity, albeit diminished. It is difficult to make a precise estimate of the risk from the hyperlipidemia because it is so commonly associated with insulin resistance or frank diabetes, which are themselves risk factors for atherosclerosis. If these are present as part of the syndrome, both CHD and peripheral arterial disease are common.

The reason why the complete absence of LPL removes the risk of atheroma is not known with certainty. It may be because:

- the incidence of diabetes is not increased in familial LPL deficiency
- fibrinogen and factor VII activity are not increased
- the conversion of VLDL and chylomicrons to the atherogenic intermediate-density lipoprotein (IDL) and remnant lipoproteins, respectively, is impaired in the absence of LPL
- serum LDL and apoB levels are decreased in familial LPL deficiency, any increase in serum cholesterol being caused by the cholesterol in VLDL and chylomicrons.

Acute pancreatitis may occur when serum triglyceride levels exceed 20–30 mmol/L (1800–2700 mg/dL). The presentation of acute pancreatitis is similar to that arising from other causes. However, increased serum amylase activity may not be present. Falsely low values may result from interference by triglyceride-rich lipoproteins in the laboratory method. All laboratories should inspect serum for milkiness (see Figure 5.1) before reporting normal or only moderately raised serum amylase activity in patients with severe abdominal pain. Clinicians may otherwise wrongly exclude the diagnosis of acute pancreatitis in favor, for example, of perforated peptic ulcer. Some patients do not develop acute pancreatitis, even when serum triglyceride levels exceed 100 mmol/L (9000 mg/dL). Others may experience recurring acute episodes.

Generally the pain subsides within a few hours or days of starting nasogastric aspiration and intravenous fluids (with nothing being taken by mouth). Pseudocysts develop occasionally if treatment is delayed. Pancreatic insufficiency may result from repeated episodes of acute pancreatitis.

Recurrent abdominal pain, not typical of pancreatitis, sometimes occurs in patients prone to marked hypertriglyceridemia. It may mimic irritable bowel syndrome. Severe abdominal pain may also be the result of splenic infarction.

Pseudohyponatremia is another complication of extreme hypertriglyceridemia, and may lead to serious consequences if unrecognized. In pseudohyponatremia, spuriously low serum sodium values are reported because much of the volume of the serum aliquot on which the sodium measurement is made is occupied by lipoproteins rather than water. When the serum triglycerides exceed 40–50 mmol/L (3600–4500 mg/dL), the concentration of sodium in the aqueous phase (and thus the serum osmolality) may be normal, while spurious serum sodium levels of 120–130 mmol/L are reported. The hazard is that these will be misinterpreted by the clinician, and a patient already seriously ill with pancreatitis, or occasionally uncontrolled diabetes, will be made more so by infusion of large volumes of isotonic saline or, worse, hypertonic saline.

Focal neurological syndromes such as hemiparesis, memory loss and loss of mental concentration may complicate extreme hypertriglyceridemia; cerebral ischemia may result from a sluggish microcirculation caused by the high concentrations of chylomicrons in the blood. Paresthesias, particularly in the feet, may also be an occasional feature, even in the absence of diabetes. Sicca syndrome and polyarthritis have also been described, but undoubtedly the most common articular association is with gout (see page 89).

Dietary modification. For patients with serum triglyceride levels exceeding 10 mmol/L (900 mg/dL), fat intake of any type must be limited; chylomicrons persisting in the fasting state will be contributing to the hypertriglyceridemia, and these are formed from any kind of dietary fat. For patients with hypertriglyceridemia who are prone to pancreatitis or who have eruptive xanthomata and hepatosplenomegaly, restriction of daily fat intake to 20 g or less may be necessary. Medium-chain triglycerides and fish oil are of no value in this situation. Carbohydrate and proteins must be substituted for fat in patients who are not obese. A dietitian attached to a specialized unit is usually best placed to give this type of advice and training.

Drug and surgical treatment. Drug therapy is generally less effective than a low-fat diet in severe hypertriglyceridemia. Fibrates or nicotinic acid can, however, be of value. In patients with recurring acute pancreatitis in whom triglyceride levels cannot be controlled, high-dose antioxidant treatment may prevent further episodes. It must, however, be admitted that the treatment of severe hypertriglyceridemia can be unsatisfactory and for obese, insulin-resistant patients experiencing recurring episodes of acute pancreatitis, pancreatico-biliary diversion has led to amelioration of diabetes, hypertriglyceridemia and attacks of pancreatitis. Similar surgical procedures in lean patients with familial LPL deficiency are much more difficult to contemplate. There is no substitute for adherence to a low-fat diet.

Key points – hypertriglyceridemia

- Severe hypertriglyceridemia increases the risk of pancreatitis.
- Moderate hypertriglyceridemia with elevated apoB increases the risk of coronary heart disease (CHD). Statins are the first-line therapy to reduce CHD risk in these patients.
- In severe hypertriglyceridemia:
  - spuriously high transaminases can make it hard to exclude liver disease
  - severe abdominal pain in the presence of milky plasma is highly likely to result from acute pancreatitis even in the absence of markedly raised amylase
  - pseudohyponatremia can confuse the clinician.

Key references

Alexandrides TK, Skroubis G, Kalfarentzos F. Resolution of diabetes mellitus and metabolic syndrome following Roux-en-Y gastric bypass and a variant of biliopancreatic diversion in patients with morbid obesity. *Obes Surg* 2007;17:176–84.

Brunzell JD, Deeb SS. Familial lipoprotein lipase deficiency, apo CII deficiency and hepatic liver deficiency. In: Scriver CR, Beaudet AL, Sly WS et al., eds. *The Metabolic and Molecular Bases of Inherited Disease*, 8th edn. New York: McGraw-Hill, 2001: 2789–816.

Durrington PN. Hypertriglyceridaemia. In: *Hyperlipidaemia: Diagnosis and Management*, 3rd edn. London: Hodder Arnold, 2007:169–202.

Heaney AP, Sharer N, Rameh B et al. Prevention of recurrent pancreatitis in familial lipoprotein lipase deficiency with high-dose antioxidant therapy. *J Clin Endocrinol Metab* 1999;84:1203–5.

Sarwar N, Danesh J, Eiriksdottir G et al. Triglycerides and the risk of coronary heart disease: 10,158 incident cases among 262,525 participants in 29 Western prospective studies. *Circulation* 2007;115:450–8.

Familial dysbetalipoproteinemia has several synonyms:

- type III hyperlipoproteinemia
- broad β disease
- floating β disease
- remnant removal disease.

It is rare, probably affecting fewer than 1 in 5000 people, and rarer still in premenopausal women and children. Familial dysbetalipoproteinemia has the distinction of being the first clinical syndrome to be associated with primary hyperlipoproteinemia, and was described by Addison (who also described adrenal insufficiency and pernicious anemia) and Gull (physician to Queen Victoria) in 1851.

The condition occurs because of the presence of increased amounts of chylomicron remnants and intermediate-density lipoprotein (or partially metabolized very-low-density lipoprotein [VLDL]), often collectively termed β-VLDL, in the circulation. This is the result of decreased clearance of these lipoproteins at the apoE (hepatic remnant; heparan sulfate/LDL receptor-related protein) receptor.

Familial dysbetalipoproteinemia undoubtedly accelerates atherosclerosis in the coronary, iliac, femoral and tibial arteries. The incidence of CHD is about the same as that in familial hypercholesterolemia (FH). Intermittent claudication, however, is much more common in familial dysbetalipoproteinemia, and is at least as frequent as coronary heart disease (CHD). In FH, peripheral arterial disease is uncommon relative to the frequency of CHD, indicating that the atherogenic process in the leg arteries is much more susceptible to the larger lipoprotein particles in familial dysbetalipoproteinemia than to the smaller low-density lipoprotein (LDL) particles in FH.

Underlying mechanism

Familial dysbetalipoproteinemia is generally an autosomal recessive condition with variable penetrance. A mutation or polymorphism of the

APOE gene appears to occur in all cases, impairing binding of apoE to its receptors. A polymorphism, apoE2, in which cysteine is substituted for arginine at position 158 (Figure 6.1), is the most common genetic association. At least 90% of patients with familial dysbetalipoproteinemia are homozygous for *APOE2*.

More often than not, however, *APOE2* homozygosity, which is present in around 1% of the population, does not itself impose such a severe strain on lipoprotein metabolism that hyperlipoproteinemia develops; this requires combination with some other disorder that causes overproduction of VLDL or some additional catabolic defect. This explains the association of familial dysbetalipoproteinemia with diabetes and hypothyroidism. More often, the additional stimulus to hyperlipoproteinemia is obesity or the co-inheritance of a polygenic tendency to hypertriglyceridemia. Rarer mutations of *APOE* have been described, including a mutation leading to apoE deficiency. These mutations behave similarly to *APOE2* homozygosity clinically, though they may not require other factors for the expression of the phenotype. Heterozygous apoE deficiency finds little clinical expression but, interestingly, rare mutations directly involving the receptor-binding domain of apoE (amino acids 124–150) produce the familial dysbetalipo-proteinemia phenotype even in heterozygotes (dominant expression), implying that such mutations are a greater handicap to receptor clearance than a mutation in one gene causing non-expression of apoE.

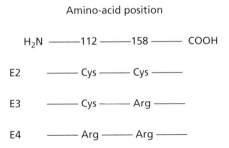

Figure 6.1 Amino-acid substitutions in the commonly occurring genetic polymorphisms of apoE (apoE2, apoE3 and apoE4). Cys, cysteine; Arg, arginine.

Diagnosis

Cholesterol and triglycerides. Serum cholesterol and fasting triglyceride concentrations are increased, typically to 7–12 mmol/L (280–480 mg/dL) for cholesterol, and to 5–20 mmol/L (450–1800 mg/dL) for triglycerides. The concentrations of cholesterol and triglycerides are often similar, and this may be a clue that a patient has familial dysbetalipoproteinemia. Another clue is that serum apoB is not elevated. The combination of a markedly elevated cholesterol and triglyceride in the face of a normal apoB should provoke serious consideration of this diagnosis. Occasionally, the condition is associated with marked hypertriglyceridemia because of overwhelming chylomicronemia. A simple diagnostic algorithm based on total cholesterol, triglyceride and apoB has been validated for all the atherogenic apoB dyslipoproteinemias.

Xanthomata are present in more than half of patients with familial dysbetalipoproteinemia. Striate palmar xanthomata (Figure 6.2) and tuberoeruptive xanthomata (Figure 6.3) are characteristic. Striate palmar xanthomata can simply be an orange discoloration of the palmar

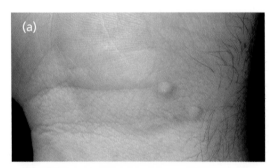

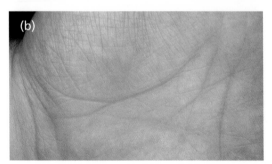

Figure 6.2 Striate palmar xanthomata (a) with some raised lesions, and (b) showing simply as an orange-yellow discoloration within the creases of the palmar skin.

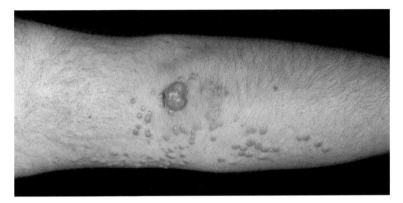

Figure 6.3 Tuberoeruptive xanthomata showing cauliflower-like tuberose deposits on the point of the elbow and eruptive satellite lesions.

skin creases. They may, however, be more florid and appear as raised, seed-like lesions (sometimes even larger) in the skin creases of the palms, fingers and flexor surfaces of the wrists. Tuberoeruptive xanthomata occur over the elbows and knees, and sometimes over other tuberosities, such as the heels and dorsum of the interphalangeal joints of the fingers. They resolve entirely with successful treatment.

Laboratory tests. The diagnosis of familial dysbetalipoproteinemia hyperlipoproteinemia is not difficult in the presence of typical xanthomata. When these are absent, laboratory tests are required. Type IIb or V hyperlipoproteinemia can give similar serum lipid levels.

Polyacrylamide gel isoelectric focusing or DNA testing by restriction-fragment-length polymorphism, available in many specialized centers, can be used to identify *APOE2* homozygosity. *APOE2* homozygosity in the presence of hyperlipidemia makes the diagnosis of familial dysbetalipoproteinemia virtually certain. When the *APOE2* homozygosity is absent in a patient with the typical familial dysbetalipoproteinemia clinical phenotype, some other *APOE* mutation is usually present. Its identification, though of great theoretical value at a specialized center, is often impossible and, fortunately, is of little practical importance.

Testing for the *APOE* genotype may reveal that a patient does not have familial dysbetalipoproteinemia, but provide the unwelcome finding that *APOE4* is present. This allele has been linked with

Alzheimer's disease – certainly in its late-onset form but also, in some studies, with the early-onset type. It is probably wise for the laboratory reporting the *APOE* genotype results to report only whether *APOE2* homozygosity is present or absent. Otherwise, information about many people's *APOE4* genotype will be gratuitously available in their medical records without their consent or any explanation to them as to the possible consequences of its knowledge.

Ultracentrifugation. If clinical diagnosis of familial dysbetalipoproteinemia requires confirmation in the absence of *APOE2* homozygosity, plasma should be sent to a center that can identify cholesterol-rich VLDL (β-VLDL) typical of dysbetalipoproteinemia using ultracentrifugation.

It is also important to exclude paraproteinemia by immunoglobulin electrophoresis. This can produce hyperlipoproteinemia mimicking familial dysbetalipoproteinemia.

Treatment

Diet. Familial dysbetalipoproteinemia can be responsive to a reduction in obesity. In the occasional lean patient, a diet in which monounsaturated and polyunsaturated fats and carbohydrates are substituted for saturated fat can be helpful unless triglycerides exceed 10 mmol/L (900 mg/dL). If this is the case, a diet low in all types of fat, with carbohydrate substitution, may be necessary.

Fibrates and statins. Familial dysbetalipoproteinemia is generally responsive to statins and fibrates. In view of the high risk of atherosclerosis it is sensible to adopt an intensive attitude to treatment and aim to achieve total serum cholesterol levels less than 4 mmol/L (160 mg/dL), and triglyceride concentrations less than 1.7 mmol/L (150 mg/dL) using, if necessary, a combination of statin and fibrate treatment. Even if after dietary modification the triglycerides remain only moderately elevated and cholesterol is at target, it is generally wise to introduce fibrate therapy, because even a moderate increase in triglycerides probably indicates that the abnormal β-VLDL is present in quantities that may still be harmful.

Key points – familial dysbetalipoproteinemia

- Peripheral vascular disease is as common as coronary heart disease in individuals with familial dysbetalipoproteinemia.
- Palmar and tuberoeruptive xanthomata are a key to diagnosis.
- Cholesterol and triglycerides are elevated, their concentrations often being similar.
- Fibrates are the first line of pharmacological therapy.

Key references

de Graaf J, Couture P, Sniderman A. A diagnostic algorithm for the atherogenic apolipoprotein B dyslipoproteinemias. *Nat Clin Pract Endocrinol Metab* 2008;4:608–18.

Durrington PN. Type III hyperlipoproteinaemia. In: *Hyperlipidaemia: Diagnosis and Management*, 3rd edn. London: Hodder Arnold, 2007:203–13.

Mahley RW, Rall SC. Type III hyperlipoproteinemia (dysbetalipoproteinemia): the role of apolipoprotein E in normal and abnormal lipoprotein metabolism. In: Scriver CR, Beaudet AL, Sly WS et al., eds. *The Metabolic and Molecular Bases of Inherited Disease*, 8th edn. New York: McGraw-Hill, 2001:2835–62.

National Institute on Ageing. The Alzheimer's Association Working Group. Apolipoprotein E genotyping in Alzheimer's disease. *Lancet* 1996; 347:1091–5.

7 Dyslipidemia in insulin resistance, the metabolic syndrome and diabetes mellitus

The dyslipidemia associated with diabetes mellitus is generally classified as a secondary hyperlipidemia. However, we have chosen to give it a chapter of its own and to deal with the other secondary hyperlipidemias in the next chapter. In part, this is because of the importance of diabetic dyslipidemia, but it is also because, increasingly, we recognize that the following features associated with type 2 diabetes often exist long before the blood glucose climbs to diabetic levels (Table 7.1):

- raised triglycerides and low high-density lipoprotein (HDL) cholesterol
- increased small, dense low-density lipoprotein (LDL) and, therefore, increased apoB
- hypertension
- most importantly, elevated cardiovascular risk.

At this earlier euglycemic stage, patients are classified not as diabetic, but as having insulin resistance or metabolic syndrome. Strictly, they have a primary dyslipidemia. Later, many become diabetic as a consequence of becoming increasingly insulin resistant (centrally obese) or being unable to maintain the high rate of insulin secretion required to maintain euglycemia in the face of insulin resistance, or both.

The pursuit of glycemic control should never be regarded as the sole aim of diabetes management, because this will do little to ameliorate the high rate of macrovascular complications associated with both type 1 and type 2 diabetes. First, bear in mind that there is, as yet, no evidence of any clear, powerful and continuous relationship between coronary risk and degree of hyperglycemia. Put differently, the diagnosis of diabetes or impaired fasting glucose substantially increases risk, whereas the degree of hyperglycemia beyond that does not. Second, though tighter glucose control reduces the incidence of microvascular disease, only modest benefit has as yet been shown regarding the risk of macrovascular disease, and some of that may be due to the lipid-lowering effects of hypoglycemic agents such as insulin and metformin. Third, it is well documented, though not widely appreciated, that the

TABLE 7.1

Risk factors for cardiovascular disease in men and women who developed diabetes in the next 8 years and in those who did not*

	Men		Women	
	Did not develop diabetes	Became diabetic	Did not develop diabetes	Became diabetic
BMI (kg/m²)	27.8	29.9	26.5	31.3
Triglycerides (mmol/L)	1.62	2.18	1.19	1.95
Cholesterol (mmol/L)	5.55	5.84	5.20	5.84
LDL-C (mmol/L)	3.65	3.90	3.25	3.87
HDL-C (mmol/L)	1.17	1.08	1.36	1.06
SBP (mmHg)	113	118	107	112
DBP (mmHg)	75	77	69	75
Fasting glucose (mmol/L)	5.15	5.68	4.94	5.51
Fasting insulin (pmol/L)	95	158	91	201

BMI, body mass index; DBP diastolic blood pressure; HD, high-density lipoprotein; LDL, low-density lipoprotein; SBP, systolic blood pressure.
*Data from Haffner SM et al. *JAMA* 1990;263:2893–8.

incidence of microvascular disease differs little among people with type 2 diabetes around the world. By contrast, the incidence of macrovascular disease differs considerably, being much higher in societies in which energy intake is excessive and a high proportion of energy intake comes from dietary fat rather than carbohydrate.

These differences in risk are most likely to relate to differences in the prevalence of the atherogenic dyslipoproteinemias and hypertension. In other words, it is dyslipoproteinemia and hypertension, rather than hyperglycemia, that are the major driving forces for vascular disease in diabetes. The clear reduction in clinical cardiovascular events produced by statin therapy supports this view incontrovertibly.

The concept of insulin resistance was introduced by Gerald Reaven. Initially, the defining abnormality was the requirement for higher concentrations of insulin to maintain normal blood glucose during insulin infusion studies; this was related to a reduction in the efficiency with which insulin produced glucose uptake in skeletal muscle. This concept was extended to adipose tissue: insulin resistance was equated with an increased release of none-esterified fatty acids (NEFA) through increased triglyceride lipolysis during fasting, which was related to a failure of insulin to suppress hormone-sensitive lipase activity. Thus, dysglycemia was linked to dyslipidemia.

The biological mechanisms of insulin 'resistance' have not been fully identified. Nevertheless, the construct has drawn powerful support as it appears to explain a variety of abnormalities that commonly coexist. These abnormalities – dysglycemia, dyslipidemia, abdominal obesity and hypertension – have been grouped into what is now defined as the metabolic syndrome. A joint interim statement from the International Diabetes Federation, American Heart Association, World Heart Federation, International Atherosclerotic Society and International Association for the Study of Obesity, published in 2009, attempted to harmonize different definitions of the metabolic syndrome, and set single cut-off points for variables (Table 7.2), with the exception of waist circumference. In the case of this last measure, the interim statement recommends that clinicians and researchers refer to national or regional recommendations for waist circumference cut-off points.

From our perspective, the major problem with the metabolic syndrome is that some of the most important features can differ in cause, consequence and therapy. In Europe and the USA, hypertriglyceridemia is most commonly caused by increased fatty-acid flux to the liver, increasing the risk of vascular disease because the concentration of small, dense LDL particles is markedly increased. In other countries where coronary heart disease (CHD) is less frequent and the diet is one in which most energy is derived from carbohydrate as opposed to fat, moderate increases in triglycerides are often not associated with raised apoB levels and increased coronary risk. Adding apoB identifies the really high-risk subgroup within the total mass of numbers of patients with the metabolic syndrome. As only a proportion of patients meeting the criteria for metabolic syndrome have an elevated apoB, measuring apoB will allow therapeutic energy to be concentrated on those who need it most.

TABLE 7.2

Criteria for the metabolic syndrome, as proposed in the joint interim statement from multiple organizations

Variable	Cut-off point
Elevated waist circumferance*	Refer to national or population cut-off points
Elevated triglycerides (drug treatment for elevated triglycerides is another indicator[†])	≥ 1.7 mmol/L (150 mg/dL)
Reduced HDL-C (drug treatment for reduced HDL-C is another indicator[†])	< 1.0 mmol/L (40 mg/dL) in men < 1.3 mmol/L (50 mg/dL) in women
Elevated blood pressure (anti-hypertensive drug treatment in a patient with a history of hypertension is another indicator)	Systolic ≥ 130 mmHg and/or diastolic ≥ 85 mmHg
Elevated fasting glucose[‡] (drug treatment for elevated glucose is another indicator)	≥ 5.5 mmol/L (100 mg/dL)

From Alberti et al. 2009.
*Until more data are available, cut-off points from the International Diabetes Federation (IDF) are recommended for non-Europeans and either the IDF or American Heart Association/National Heart, Lung, and Blood Institute cut-off points for people of European origin.
[†]The most commonly used drugs for elevated triglycerides and reduced HDL-C are fibrates and nicotinic acid. A patient taking one of these drugs can be presumed to have high triglycerides and low HDL-C. High-dose ω-3 fatty acids presumes high triglycerides.
[‡]Most patients with type 2 diabetes mellitus will have the metabolic syndrome.
HDL-C, high-density lipoprotein cholesterol.

Hypertriglyceridemia

Hypertriglyceridemia is the dominant hyperlipidemia in diabetes. Moderately raised triglyceride levels are common, and occasionally severe hypertriglyceridemia occurs, sometimes to levels in excess of 100 mmol/L (9000 mg/dL), leading to the development of eruptive xanthomata and occasionally other features of the chylomicronemia syndrome. Lipemia retinalis can interfere with laser photocoagulation therapy for diabetic retinopathy. Lipoprotein lipase (LPL) is activated by insulin. Thus, its activity is diminished with the insulin deficiency and/or resistance associated with uncontrolled diabetes. For severe hypertriglyceridemia to occur, there is generally an additional fault in triglyceride metabolism that predisposes the patient to hypertriglyceridemia. Often, this predisposing factor is a mutation in one of the LPL genes, leading to a defect in triglyceride catabolism which, in the absence of diabetes, might produce only a modest rise in triglycerides. Less often, tuberoeruptive xanthomata and striate palmar xanthomata indicate that florid familial dysbetalipoproteinemia has occurred in a genetically susceptible individual (usually an *APOE2* homozygote).

In most patients with diabetes whose glycemia is under reasonable control, any persisting hypertriglyceridemia is not caused by a major defect in triglyceride catabolism, but by overproduction of very-low-density lipoprotein (VLDL) by the liver. NEFA arriving at the liver from the adipose tissue in increased quantities is likely to be a major reason for increased hepatic triglyceride synthesis and VLDL secretion. NEFA is released in increased quantities from adipose tissue when the quantity of adipose tissue is increased (i.e. in obesity), which often occurs in type 2 diabetes mellitus. In diabetes, triglyceride release from the liver is further facilitated by decreased insulin secretion and/or insulin resistance, which will decrease the direct inhibitory effect of insulin on the secretion of VLDL by hepatocytes. Even in insulin-treated diabetes, the liver is likely to remain deficient in insulin because insulin administered via the subcutaneous route arrives at the liver from the systemic circulation rather than via the portal vein: physiologically, the concentration of insulin in the portal circulation is several times that in the systemic circulation. To achieve such high portal insulin levels by systemic administration of insulin would subject peripheral tissues to grossly supraphysiological levels.

Patients with type 1 diabetes mellitus are less likely to have hypertriglyceridemia than those with type 2 diabetes. This may be partly because insulin therapy is the rule in type 1 diabetes, and also because other factors predisposing to hypertriglyceridemia, such as obesity, and β-blocker and diuretic therapies, are more common in people with type 2 diabetes. There may, however, be a more fundamental reason. Free fatty acids are disposed of by the liver in three major processes:

- complete oxidation
- partial oxidation (ketogenesis)
- esterification (triglyceride synthesis).

When hepatic energy requirements are met, only ketogenesis and esterification are possible. In type 2 diabetes, NEFA are not readily converted to ketone bodies for reasons not entirely understood, whereas in type 1 diabetes their entry into the mitochondria, where β-oxidation occurs, is facilitated. Resistance to ketogenesis in type 2 diabetes may thus carry with it a predisposition to hypertriglyceridemia.

There may also be a defect in the regulation of postprandial lipoprotein metabolism in diabetes. Normally, the burst of insulin secretion that immediately follows a meal inhibits hepatic VLDL secretion and promotes hepatic triglyceride storage. This relieves pressure on the triglyceride catabolic pathways, allowing more rapid chylomicron clearance. Later, when insulin levels decline, hepatic VLDL secretion increases and stored triglycerides are mobilized. In diabetes, failure to suppress VLDL secretion following meals occurs because of insulin resistance or deficiency, leading to high levels of remnant particles and intermediate-density lipoprotein (IDL) in the circulation.

The triglyceride-rich lipoproteins are not themselves directly responsible for the increased atherogenic risk. Rather, the culprits are the smaller, lipid-poor lipoproteins produced by their catabolism. These include increased quantities of small, dense LDL as well as increased numbers of remnant particles. Lower HDL also increases risk.

Serum LDL cholesterol and apoB levels

LDL cholesterol is a poor marker for LDL particle number in patients with type 2 diabetes. Typical results for a group of 249 adults with type 2 diabetes are shown in Table 7.3, which lists the average levels for each parameter as well as the percentile of the population with which the value accords. It is evident that total and LDL cholesterol are normal, triglycerides elevated and HDL cholesterol decreased. The level of small, dense LDL is elevated. Note that the apoB is high (70th percentile) compared with the LDL cholesterol (50th percentile).

Figure 7.1 shows two ways of dividing the overall group into phenotypes: the first based on triglyceride and LDL cholesterol, the

TABLE 7.3

Lipid and apoB levels in individuals with type 2 diabetes (n = 249)*

	Mean value	Percentile of normal population
Age	59 years	
Total serum cholesterol	5.34 mmol/L (205 mg/dL)	~ 50th
Total serum triglycerides	2.13 mmol/L (189 mg/dL)	~ 60th
LDL cholesterol	3.28 mmol/L (126 mg/dL)	~ 50th
apoB	114 mg/dL	~ 70th
HDL cholesterol	1.12 mmol/L (43 mg/dL)	~ 35th

HDL, high-density lipoprotein; LDL, low-denisty lipoprotein.
*Data from Sniderman AD et al. *Diabetes Care* 2002;25:579–82.

second on triglyceride and apoB. Note that in the first, only about 20% of patients have an elevated LDL cholesterol. By contrast, about 40% have an elevated LDL particle number based on apoB. Even though apoB testing is not available to most clinicians, knowledge of the underlying increase in apoB, small, dense LDL and IDL helps to explain the benefit of statin and gemfibrozil therapy in diabetes evident in the studies HPS, 4S, CARE, LIPID, CARDS, ASCOT and VA-HIT. In neither FIELD, in which fenofibrate was tested as a single agent in patients with type 2 diabetes, nor in ACCORD, in which the combination of fenofibrate and statin versus statin alone was tested in patients with type 2 diabetes, was the primary endpoint achieved. These results mean that fibrates cannot be recommended to lower cardiovascular risk in patients with diabetes.

Serum HDL cholesterol concentrations tend to be low in type 2 diabetes, whereas in type 1 they are normal or even raised. The low levels in type 2 diabetes are largely explained by the presence of associated hypertriglyceridemia, obesity, cigarette smoking, abstention from alcohol, raised cholesteryl ester transfer protein activity and low LPL activity and the use of drugs such as β-blockers. These factors are

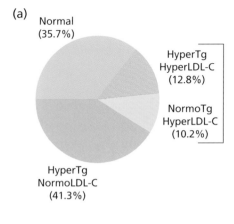

(a)

Normal
(35.7%)

HyperTg
HyperLDL-C
(12.8%)

NormoTg
HyperLDL-C
(10.2%)

HyperTg
NormoLDL-C
(41.3%)

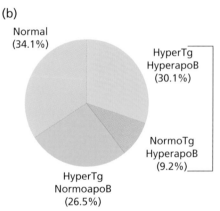

(b)

Normal
(34.1%)

HyperTg
HyperapoB
(30.1%)

NormoTg
HyperapoB
(9.2%)

HyperTg
NormoapoB
(26.5%)

Figure 7.1 Two ways of dividing a group of 249 individuals with type 2 diabetes into lipid-level phenotypes: (a) based on serum triglyceride (Tg) and low-density lipoprotein cholesterol (LDL-C); (b) based on serum triglycerides and apolipoprotein B (apoB). Only 23% have elevated LDL cholesterol, but 39% have elevated apoB.

less common in type 1 diabetes, and some other influence – probably insulin therapy – tends to increase HDL. A possible mechanism is that insulin increases HDL as a result of stimulating LPL activity. The raised HDL cholesterol in type 1 diabetes is not as protective against atheroma as would be expected in the absence of diabetes, probably because it has a diminished capacity to protect LDL against oxidative modification.

Effect of hypoglycemic drugs

Improving glycemic control generally has a beneficial effect on lipoproteins. Metformin also has an independent lipid-lowering action. Unfortunately, sulfonylurea and thiazolidinediones are associated with body weight gain, which may overwhelm any favorable effects they may have. Insulin too, though its action is to lower triglycerides and cholesterol and raise HDL, may stimulate weight gain and thus increase insulin resistance, again nullifying or even reversing any beneficial effects.

Proteinuria, hypertension and hyperfibrinogenemia

These often coexist with hyperlipidemia in diabetes and increase coronary risk considerably. Nephropathy, as in the case of primary renal disease, may exacerbate hyperlipoproteinemia. Furthermore, proteinuria in diabetes indicates a generalized increase in vascular permeability, and thus macromolecules such as LDL may enter the arterial subintima at increased rates – an effect aided and abetted by hypertension.

Abnormal serum liver function tests and fatty liver

These occur commonly in diabetes and insulin resistance (see the section on liver disease in Chapter 8).

Key points – dyslipidemia in insulin resistance, the metabolic syndrome and diabetes mellitus

- Dyslipidemia is an integral element of type 1 and type 2 diabetes and their associated vascular risk.
- Statins are the first line of therapy for diabetic dyslipidemias unless hypertriglyceridemia is particularly marked.
- Once statin treatment has been instituted, treatment of persisting hypertriglyceridemia is controversial, but undoubtedly fibrates are being used less commonly (see Chapter 5).

Key references

Alberti KGMM, Eckel RH, Grundy SM et al. Harmonizing the metabolic syndrome: a Joint Interim Statement of the International Diabetes Federation Task Force on Epidemiology and Prevention; National Heart, Lung, and Blood Institute; American Heart Association; World Heart Federation; International Atherosclerosis Society; and International Association for the Study of Obesity. *Circulation* 2009;120;1640–45.

Buse JB, Ginsberg HN, Bakris GL et al. Primary prevention of cardiovascular disease in people with diabetes mellitus. A scientific statement from the American Heart Association and the American Diabetes Association. *Circulation* 2007;115:114–26.

Durrington PN, Charlton-Menys V. Diabetic dyslipidaemia. In: Barnett AH, ed. *Diabetes – Best Practice & Research Compendium*. London: Elsevier, 2006:157–67.

Haffner SM, Stern MP, Hazuda HP et al. Cardiovascular risk factors in confirmed prediabetic individuals: does the clock for coronary disease start ticking before the onset of clinical diabetes? *JAMA* 1990; 263:2893–8.

Howard BV, Robbins DC, Sievers ML et al. LDL cholesterol as a strong predictor of coronary heart disease in diabetic individuals with insulin resistance and low LDL: the Strong Heart Study. *Arterioscler Thromb Vasc Biol* 2000;20:830–5.

Kuller LH, Velentgas P, Barzilay J et al. Diabetes mellitus: subclinical cardiovascular disease and risk of incident cardiovascular disease and all-cause mortality. *Arterioscler Thromb Vasc Biol* 2000;20:823–9.

Lean MEJ. Obesity and eating disorders. In: Betteridge DJ, Illingworth DR, Shepherd J, eds. *Lipoproteins in Health and Disease*. London: Arnold, 1999:881–95.

Reaven G. Metabolic syndrome: pathophysiology and implications for management of cardiovascular disease. *Circulation* 2002;106:286–8.

Ryden L, Standl E, Bartnik M et al. Task Force on Diabetes and Cardiovascular Diseases of the European Society of Cardiology (ESC); European Association for the Study of Diabetes (EASD). Guidelines on diabetes, pre-diabetes, and cardiovascular diseases: executive summary. *Eur Heart J* 2007;28: 88–136.

Scobie IN, Samaras K. *Fast Facts: Diabetes mellitus*, 3rd edn. Oxford: Health Press Ltd, 2009.

Hyperlipidemia commonly coexists with other diseases. These diseases may be the complications of the hyperlipidemia, such as coronary heart disease (CHD) or pancreatitis; sometimes, however, it is the hyperlipidemia which is the complication of another disease. In this case, the dyslipidemia represents a secondary rather than a primary derangement of lipoprotein metabolism. Hyperlipidemia may also be associated with another disorder more commonly than would be expected by chance alone, such as gout, even though there is no known metabolic link.

The secondary hyperlipidemias (Table 8.1) are important because:
- the secondary hyperlipidemia may be a cause of morbidity
- the hyperlipidemia may accelerate the progress of the primary disease, as has been suggested to be the case in renal and liver disease.

Table 8.2 shows the effect on serum lipoprotein levels of some dyslipidemias generally regarded as secondary. (Type 1 and type 2 diabetes are the subject of Chapter 7; please see our comments about type 2 diabetes at the beginning of the previous chapter.)

Obesity

The overall relation of obesity to the risk of cardiovascular disease is not strong. However, if cases are divided into those with abdominal versus peripheral obesity, risk is high for the former but not for the latter. In abdominal obesity, hypertriglyceridemia with elevated apoB is frequent, whereas in peripheral obesity it is not.

Sex plays a major role in the pathophysiology of the two forms of obesity. Abdominal obesity is so common in males that the pattern is called android obesity. By contrast, peripheral obesity is common in females, and this pattern is designated gynecoid obesity. The insulin resistance it produces is the consequence of the high rate of free fatty acid release from this type of adipose tissue. Also, the various chemokines and inflammatory cytokines it releases contribute to the insulin resistance and vascular risk.

TABLE 8.1

Diseases and physiological or pharmacological perturbations associated with hyperlipidemia

Endocrine
- Diabetes mellitus
- Thyroid disease
- Pituitary disease
- Pregnancy

Renal disease
- Nephrotic syndrome
- Chronic renal failure

Drugs
- β-blockers
- Thiazide diuretics
- Steroid hormones
- Microsomal enzyme-inducing agents (e.g. phenytoin, phenobarbital, griseofulvin)
- Retinoic-acid derivatives (e.g. isotretinoin)
- HIV antiretroviral therapy

Hepatic disease
- Cholestasis
- Hepatocellular disease
- Cholelithiasis

Immunoglobulin excess
- Myeloma
- Macroglobulinemia
- Systemic lupus erythematosus

Hyperuricemia

Miscellaneous
- Glycogen storage disease
- Lipodystrophies

Nutritional
- Obesity
- Alcohol
- Anorexia nervosa

A number of investigators have proposed that such patients be identified on the basis of elevated triglycerides and increased waist circumference – the so-called 'hypertriglyceridemic waist syndrome'. These patients have higher insulin and apoB levels. Measuring apoB is a more direct and accurate way to assess risk but, in its absence, this alternative approach is useful.

Thyroid disease

Serum low-density lipoprotein (LDL) cholesterol and, more rarely, serum triglycerides are raised in hypothyroidism. Receptor-mediated

TABLE 8.2

Lipoprotein levels associated with various conditions

Cause	VLDL	LDL	HDL
Type 1 diabetes	↑	– or ↓	– or ↑
Type 2 diabetes	↑↑	↑	↓
Hypothyroidism	↑	↑↑	↑
Pregnancy	↑	↑	↑
Obesity	↑	– or ↑	↓
Alcohol	↑	– or ↑	↑
Nephrotic syndrome	↑	↑↑	– or ↓
Chronic renal failure	↑	–	↓
Cholestasis	–	↑↑ (LpX)	↓
Hepatocellular disease	↑ (IDL)	–	↓
Hyperuricemia	↑	–	↓

HDL, high-density lipoprotein; IDL, intermediate-density lipoprotein; LDL, low-density lipoprotein; LpX, lipoprotein X; VLDL, very-low-density lipoprotein.

LDL catabolism is decreased; triglyceride catabolism and lipoprotein lipase (LPL) activity may also be reduced. High-density lipoprotein (HDL) levels also tend to be increased because of diminished transfer of cholesteryl ester to other lipoproteins. These effects may be reversible with thyroxine replacement (Figure 8.1), which also restores biliary cholesterol excretion to normal from a depressed level.

Subclinical hypothyroidism – that is, raised serum thyroid-stimulating hormone (TSH), but thyroxine in the normal range – may influence serum LDL slightly. In one survey, serum TSH was raised in 20% of women over the age of 40 years with serum cholesterol exceeding 8 mmol/L (320 mg/dL). Although only 5% were actually hypothyroid, findings such as these underline the importance of adequately excluding hypothyroidism in those with hypercholesterolemia beyond midlife.

Hyperthyroidism. There is a tendency towards decreased LDL and HDL cholesterol in hyperthyroidism, but hypertriglyceridemia can occur.

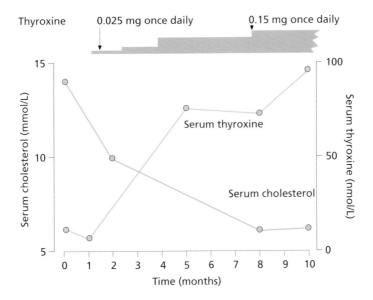

Figure 8.1 Effect of thyroxine-replacement therapy on serum cholesterol in a patient with hypothyroidism.

Renal disease

Nephrotic syndrome. When proteinuria occurs in patients with relatively normal creatinine clearance, the predominant effect is to increase LDL (either from increased production of very-low-density lipoprotein (VLDL) or by an increase in the amount of LDL directly secreted by the liver), thus producing hypercholesterolemia. The severity of the hypercholesterolemia is often proportional to the decrease in serum albumin.

Hypertriglyceridemia in nephrotic syndrome is unusual in the absence of hypercholesterolemia; it is more likely where chronic renal failure is also present, when it is often associated with decreased LPL. VLDL secretion by cultured hepatocytes decreases in response to albumin or other macromolecules introduced into the culture medium; the intravenous infusion of albumin or other macromolecules into patients with nephrotic syndrome reduces LDL levels. Both effects may be caused by changes in osmotic pressure or viscosity.

85

Serum HDL cholesterol levels are usually normal or decreased in nephrotic syndrome. Even when total HDL is normal, there is a shift towards smaller particles, so that the less dense HDL2 subfraction decreases while the more dense HDL3 often increases. Loss of HDL from the circulation increases because of leakage from the kidney, and this is related to the selectivity and extent of the glomerular leak. Immunoreactive apoAI in quantities equal to the normal daily apoAI production may be found in the urine; to maintain relatively normal serum HDL cholesterol levels, HDL production is greatly increased in many patients with proteinuria.

Chronic renal failure without proteinuria is characterized by hypertriglyceridemia. Both VLDL and LDL are enriched with triglycerides in patients with renal failure. However, apoB is normal to low. There is also a tendency for remnant particles to persist in the circulation. The underlying cause is uncertain, but it may relate to decreased activity of both LPL and hepatic lipase. Insulin resistance associated with renal failure does not appear to increase none-esterified fatty-acid flux as it often does in other conditions. Hemodialysis further exacerbates hypertriglyceridemia; heparin depletes LPL and, in addition, there is loss of apoCII, the activator of LPL, from the circulation.

Evidence that statins decrease CHD risk in patients with end-stage renal disease is currently lacking, but statins undoubtedly lower risk in moderate renal impairment and after transplantation. Chronic ambulatory peritoneal dialysis leads to the absorption of considerable amounts of glucose from the peritoneum, producing obesity and exacerbating hypertriglyceridemia. In addition, LDL apoB is often raised, even when LDL cholesterol levels are not.

Serum HDL cholesterol levels are low in patients with chronic renal failure, whereas serum levels of lipoprotein (a) (Lp[a]) are often markedly elevated in all types of renal disease. Lp(a) comprises an LDL-like particle that contains apo(a) in addition to the usual apoB. Apo(a) is encoded by a member of the plasminogen supergene family and has much structural similarity with plasminogen. It appears to be an independent risk factor for CHD and cerebrovascular disease when present in high concentrations. Whether increased Lp(a) contributes to heightened susceptibility to atherosclerosis in renal disease is currently uncertain.

Many of the lipoprotein abnormalities resolve following renal transplantation if good renal function is established. However, hyperlipidemia persists in about one-quarter of patients, perhaps because of corticosteroid therapy, weight gain, antihypertensive therapy and, possibly, ciclosporin treatment.

Alcohol

Alcoholic beverages, particularly beer and wine, are energy rich and may be a cause of obesity. In addition, alcohol itself affects lipoprotein metabolism. Its dominant effect is to produce hypertriglyceridemia by increasing hepatic triglyceride synthesis. In turn, this leads to increased VLDL secretion. Fatty liver ensues if the mechanism for VLDL assembly and secretion fails to keep pace with production of triglyceride. Usually, alcohol overindulgence produces type IV hyperlipoproteinemia, but in individuals with a constitutional tendency to delayed triglyceride catabolism a spectacular type V hyperlipoproteinemia may occur; this may be one explanation for the association between alcohol consumption and acute pancreatitis.

Serum LDL cholesterol levels tend to be low and HDL cholesterol raised in chronic alcoholics, unless liver disease has developed. The effect on HDL is evident in moderate drinkers, mainly because of an effect on smaller HDL particles (HDL3). In heavy drinkers, larger HDL2 particles contribute more to any increase in HDL.

Recognizing occult alcoholism is obviously important, particularly in hypertriglyceridemic patients prone to pancreatitis. Measuring serum γ-glutamyl transpeptidase is not always helpful in identifying patients who drink heavily, because it may be raised in patients with hypertriglyceridemia unrelated to alcohol.

Liver disease

Cholestasis. Hypercholesterolemia occurs in obstructive jaundice without severe hepatocellular dysfunction. This is because there is an increase in unesterified cholesterol in lipoprotein particles of hydrated density similar to that of LDL (see over). Moderate hypertriglyceridemia and an increase in the plasma phospholipid lecithin (phosphatidylcholine) may also occur.

The lipoproteins of density similar to LDL are not true apoB-containing LDL, levels of which may be low, but are predominantly another lipoprotein, designated lipoprotein X (LpX). This contains unesterified cholesterol and phospholipid in an approximately equal molar ratio. LpX has a lamellar structure and on electron microscopy appears as stacks of disk-like vesicles. LpX comprises 6% protein, of which at least half is albumin enclosed within the vesicles. Apolipoproteins, particularly the apoCs, are present on its surface. Biliary cholesterol contributes to the cholesterol of LpX, but diversion of this from the obstructed biliary tree back into the circulation is, on its own, insufficient to explain the extent of the hypercholesterolemia that occurs in many patients. Decreased lecithin-cholesterol acyl transferase (LCAT) activity (see page 16) also contributes to the accumulation of unesterified cholesterol, but again this is unlikely to be the sole cause of the hypercholesterolemia because only relatively small quantities of LpX are formed when LCAT activity is even more profoundly decreased in familial LCAT deficiency. In patients with biliary obstruction, LpX in the blood appears to result largely from the reflux into the circulation of biliary phospholipids, which attract cholesterol out of cell membranes.

LpX is catabolized by the reticuloendothelial system, including the Kupffer cells. Although it is not itself taken up by the hepatocyte, LpX may interfere with hepatic uptake of chylomicron remnants. The emerging view is that a system may exist for the sequestration of remnants in the space of Disse before uptake by the hepatocyte; it is interesting to speculate that this may be a site of their interaction with LpX. This may explain the persistence of remnant-like lipoproteins in patients with obstructive jaundice.

Hepatocellular disease is often accompanied by moderate hypertriglyceridemia, reflecting the presence of triglyceride-rich lipoproteins with density in the VLDL and LDL range. The HDL consists predominantly of small particles. The accumulation of small HDL and the decrease in cholesteryl ester is secondary to LCAT deficiency, and the lipoproteins intermediate between VLDL and LDL probably build up because of hepatic lipase deficiency and other damage to the remnant-removal mechanism.

In addition to dyslipidemia caused by hepatocellular disease, dyslipidemia (or at least the obesity and insulin resistance with which it is so commonly associated) is frequently the cause of fatty liver (hepatic steatosis). This can result in raised serum γ-glutamyl transpeptidase and transaminase levels even in the absence of excessive alcohol consumption (non-alcoholic steatohepatitis or NASH). Because such patients are often at high cardiovascular risk, deciding whether to treat their dyslipidemia with lipid-lowering medications, such as statins or fibrates, which could potentially exacerbate liver disease, is a common problem. Generally, when alkaline phosphatase is not elevated and transaminase levels are no more than twice the upper limit of normal, confirmation that fatty liver is the only diagnosis can be inferred from abdominal ultrasound combined with serological exclusion of a viral or immunologic cause and careful enquiry about excessive alcohol intake. Liver biopsy is reserved for those in whom a cause other than NASH is still suspected or in whom there is concern that NASH may have progressed to cirrhosis. In patients in whom NASH is considered to be the diagnosis, lipid-lowering therapy may be used with careful monitoring of transaminase levels.

Hyperuricemia and gout

Hyperuricemia is present in a high proportion (probably half or more) of men with hypertriglyceridemia. As a result, gout commonly presents in patients with hypertriglyceridemia, particularly when hyperuricemia has been further 'precipitated' by thiazide diuretic administration.

The reason for the association is not entirely clear, as it appears to be more common than might be explained by the frequent coincidence of factors, such as obesity and high alcohol consumption, with hypertriglyceridemia.

Hypertriglyceridemia and hyperuricemia are not causally related, as lowering uric acid with allopurinol does not affect triglyceride levels; likewise, with two exceptions, lipid-lowering drug therapy does not alter the serum urate concentration. The two exceptions are nicotinic acid, which raises urate, and fenofibrate, which lowers it. The latter effect, however, is not mediated through the triglyceride-lowering action of fenofibrate, but through an independent uricosuric effect. Both urate and triglyceride levels may decrease on a weight-reducing diet, suggesting that they may both be epiphenomena of some underlying nutritional process. It has been suggested that dietary carbohydrate is important. Dietary fructose, which is taken up almost exclusively by the liver, induces hypertriglyceridemia and also increases urate levels, probably by diverting energy away from the hepatic urate-scavenging pathway into fructose phosphorylation.

Drugs

A large number of drugs in common use affect serum lipoprotein concentrations (Table 8.3). Those most commonly encountered in the lipid clinic are diuretics and β-blockers.

Thiazide diuretics raise VLDL and LDL by mechanisms that have not been elucidated. Their effect is generally small, but it may be more substantial in diabetes, which they also exacerbate. Diuretics do not alter HDL levels.

TABLE 8.3

Drugs affecting lipoprotein metabolism

Drug	VLDL	LDL	HDL
Thiazides	↑	↑	–
β-blockers without ISA	↑	–	↓
Estrogens	↑	– or ↓*	↑
Progestogens	–	↑	↓
Androgens	↓	↑	↓
Glucocorticoids	– or ↑	↑	↑
Hepatic microsomal enzyme-inducing agents (e.g. pheno-barbital, rifampicin, griseofulvin)	–†	–†	↑
Retinoic-acid derivatives (e.g. isotretinoin)	↑	–	–

*Decreased LDL in postmenopausal women.
† May be an unsustained increase.
  HDL, high-density lipoprotein; ISA, intrinsic sympathomimetic activity;
  LDL, low-density lipoprotein; VLDL, very-low-density lipoprotein.

β-blockers, regardless of cardioselectivity, tend to increase serum triglyceride concentrations by an effect on VLDL, and decrease HDL cholesterol. There is no convincing evidence that they affect total cholesterol or LDL cholesterol. Their effect on serum triglycerides may be marked in patients with pre-existing hypertriglyceridemia. A decrease in the clearance of triglyceride-rich lipoproteins appears to be the mechanism, perhaps resulting from a direct effect reducing the activity of LPL, or from diversion of blood flow away from the vascular bed of muscle, a site rich in the enzyme.

β-blockers with intrinsic sympathomimetic activity (ISA) have little or no effect on serum HDL and triglycerides. Of this class, pindolol has the highest ISA, but has found little favor as an antihypertensive and is unsuitable for the management of angina. Acebutolol and oxprenolol, with ISA about half that of pindolol but about double that of other β-blockers, may be valuable in some patients with hypertriglyceridemia when β-blocker therapy cannot be avoided. Labetalol, which combines α- and β-blocking activity, is reported to have little effect on serum lipoproteins.

Many reports suggest that α-blockers, calcium-channel antagonist vasodilators, direct-acting vasodilators and angiotensin-converting-enzyme inhibitors are either without effect on serum lipoproteins or may even have apparently favorable effects, such as raising HDL cholesterol. There is, however, no evidence as yet that pharmacologically induced changes of this type significantly alter disease morbidity or mortality.

Estrogens tend to raise the serum triglyceride level because of increased hepatic VLDL production. Occasionally, their administration in women with pre-existing hypertriglyceridemia has led to gross hyperchylomicronemia and consequent acute pancreatitis. In most women, the increase in triglycerides is small. Paradoxically, improvement has been reported in women with familial dysbetalipoproteinemia, possibly because estrogen induction of hepatic remnant removal outweighs any deleterious effect of increased VLDL production.

Estrogens also raise serum HDL cholesterol concentrations and, in postmenopausal women, decrease serum LDL cholesterol. However, the proportion of small, dense LDL will increase because of the hypertriglyceridemia they also produce. Moreover, there is evidence that unopposed estrogen therapy will lead to an increase in apoB in those with hypertriglyceridemia, thus producing a substantial increase in the absolute numbers of small, dense LDL particles. Estrogen also raises C-reactive protein. Whether these effects in some way explain the overall neutral or slightly adverse clinical impact of estrogens on vascular events is not certain. It is clear, however, that estrogens do not offer any substantial benefit in terms of reducing the risk of vascular disease in postmenopausal women and that we should be more cautious in the future about accepting similar claims for other agents based on surrogate outcomes.

Androgens generally cause the opposite effects to those achieved with estrogens: a decrease in serum HDL cholesterol and VLDL and an increase in LDL.

Progestogens increase LDL and decrease HDL – the strength of the effect depends on their androgenicity.

HIV antiretroviral therapy, particularly ritonavir, commonly produces combined hyperlipidemia with an elevated apoB. The effect is caused by an increased VLDL secretion which, in turn, is the consequence of therapy-induced reduced fatty-acid-trapping capacity by adipose tissue. It is daunting to consider adding yet another medication – statins – to the already too long list of drug therapies these patients must consume. However, the better the prognosis becomes in terms of reversing immunosuppression, the more important the treatment of this potentially atherogenic dyslipoproteinemia.

Other drugs. Many drugs other than those discussed above affect lipoprotein metabolism (e.g. retinoic-acid derivatives used in dermatology). Also important, because of the high rate of atherosclerosis in recipients of renal transplants, are the corticosteroids and ciclosporin used as immunosuppressive agents. Of great theoretical interest are drugs and chemicals that induce hepatic cytochrome P450, because of an associated increase in serum HDL levels. Such drugs include phenytoin, phenobarbital, rifampicin (rifampin) and griseofulvin. Chlorinated pesticides, such as lindane and DDT, have the same effect.

Key points – secondary hyperlipidemia

- When evaluating patients with dyslipidemia, consider the possibility that this feature is secondary to other diseases.
- Secondary dyslipidemia may contribute to the complications of the disease causing it.
- Statins may be prescribed in renal disease.

Key references

Anonymous. Unintended serum lipid level changes induced by some commonly used drugs. *Drug Ther Perspect* 2001;17:11–15.

Baraona E, Lieber CS. Alcohol. In: Betteridge DJ, Illingworth DR, Shepherd J, eds. *Lipoproteins in Health and Disease*. London: Arnold, 1999:1011–36.

Durrington PN. Secondary hyperlipidaemia. In: *Hyperlipidaemia: Diagnosis and Management*, 3rd edn. London: Hodder Arnold, 2007:310–59.

Edwards CM, Stacpoole PW. Rare secondary dyslipidaemias. In: Betteridge DJ, Illingworth DR, Shepherd J, eds. *Lipoproteins in Health and Disease*. London: Arnold, 1999:1069–98.

Kissebah AH, Krakower GR. Endocrine disorders. In: Betteridge DJ, Illingworth DR, Shepherd J, eds. *Lipoproteins in Health and Disease*. London: Arnold, 1999:931–41.

Miller JP. Liver disease. In: Betteridge DJ, Illingworth DR, Shepherd J, eds. *Lipoproteins in Health and Disease*. London: Arnold, 1999:985–1009.

Miller JP. Serum triglycerides, the liver and the pancreas. *Curr Opin Lipidol* 2000;11:377–82.

Muller-Wieland D, Krone W. Drug-induced effects. In: Betteridge DJ, Illingworth DR, Shepherd J, eds. *Lipoproteins in Health and Disease*. London: Arnold, 1999:1037–48.

Short CD, Durrington PN. Renal disorders. In: Betteridge DJ, Illingworth DR, Shepherd J, eds. *Lipoproteins in Health and Disease*. London: Arnold, 1999:943–66.

Recent criticisms leveled at the effectiveness of dietary treatment mostly stem from overviews of the effect of diet on lowering serum cholesterol in clinical trials. There is no doubt that clinical trials of diet are difficult to design and execute. Nevertheless, in practice, some people achieve a worthwhile reduction in cholesterol with dietary advice, and it is cheap to implement in comparison with drug treatment.

Diet can decrease both cholesterol and triglyceride levels and can significantly improve glycemic control in diabetes, sometimes even rendering the patient non-diabetic. The overviews of trials in which cardiovascular disease (CVD) incidence was the outcome measure also show that CVD risk can be diminished with diet. The fear of those critical of dietary treatment is that it may be employed as a sole means of therapy in high-risk patients who might otherwise derive considerable benefit from drug therapy. Diet should be regarded as an adjunct to lipid-lowering drug therapy in patients at high risk of a coronary event, such as those with established CVD. It should be part of the general lifestyle advice given to lower-risk patients for whom lipid-lowering drug therapy is not justified (see Chapter 10).

Failure of dietary modification to decrease cholesterol or apoB below some arbitrary level is not in itself an indication for lipid-lowering drug therapy; generally the need for drug therapy is determined by CVD risk. It is sometimes questioned whether it is worth bothering with diet in high-risk patients when the statins, for example, can produce a much more substantial decrease in serum cholesterol. The reason for continuing to advocate dietary advice is that the decrease in CVD incidence in many dietary trials was apparently greater than would have been expected from the decrease in serum cholesterol achieved in the trials. It seems, therefore, that there may be some additional beneficial effects that patients relying exclusively on pharmacological measures are denied. Not to emphasize diet in CVD prevention is to broadcast the wrong message to the public and to those responsible for determining nutritional policy.

Dietary advice should be offered to most people whose serum cholesterol exceeds 5.0 mmol/L (200 mg/dL). General advice is probably of limited value if the cholesterol is substantially higher or there is concern about CVD risk. Referral to a dietitian or to a nurse who has trained in dietary counseling is then generally advisable. If the patient does not do the cooking in the household, whoever cooks should also be present on such a visit. The importance of such a referral is that a personal dietary history will be taken so that advice can be tailored to the patient's own dietary preferences.

There are two essential components to dietary management of dyslipidemia: weight loss and reduction of saturated fat intake. These, together with salt restriction, constitute the nutritional approach to CVD prevention.

Weight reduction

Obesity is clearly related to hypercholesterolemia, hypertriglyceridemia, hyperapoB, low high-density lipoprotein cholesterol (Figure 9.1), high blood pressure, insulin resistance and diabetes mellitus. The obese patient should be advised to lose weight. Even reduction of moderate obesity is sometimes helpful. Failure to lose weight complicates the management of hyperlipidemia, hypertension and diabetes.

The best way to lose weight is to eat less, particularly fat. A consistent weight loss of about 1 lb/week (0.45 kg/week) is a very laudable target for weight reduction. Exercise cannot substitute for a reduced energy intake, except in unusual cases, but it may be critical in maintaining the decreased body weight achieved by dietary restriction. Claims that exercise alone can produce weight loss are generally based on calculations that neglect to subtract the energy expenditure of whatever else the patient would have been doing had he or she not been exercising.

Reducing saturated fat intake

The second important element of dietary modification involves decreasing saturated fat intake. Saturated fats in the diet increase both serum cholesterol and triglyceride levels; replacing them with carbohydrates (other than simple sugars and syrup), polyunsaturated

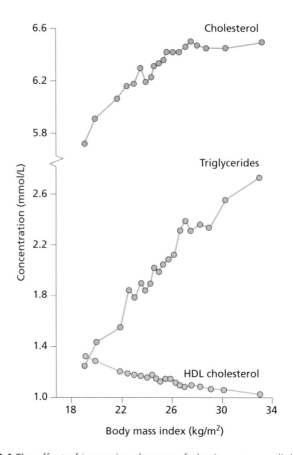

Figure 9.1 The effect of increasing degrees of obesity on serum lipids and high-density lipoprotein cholesterol. Reproduced, with permission from the BMJ Publishing Group, from Thelle et al. *Br Heart J* 1983;49:205–13.

fats or monounsaturated fats lowers the serum cholesterol and triglyceride levels. In the non-obese, in whom an energy deficit is not needed, a traditional north European and North American diet can be modified by:

- increasing the intake of potatoes, pulses, rice, pasta and fish
- using olive-oil products, and soybean, sunflower, safflower, corn or rapeseed (canola) oils.

The exception to this are patients with severe hypertriglyceridemia in whom all fats and oils should be avoided (see page 63).

Other dietary advice

Plant sterols and stanols decrease serum cholesterol and enriched margarines, yoghurt and milk are available. Those trying to lose weight should be careful that consuming these products does not increase their dietary energy intake, but otherwise they may confer some benefit, though nowhere near as much as a statin.

Fruit and vegetables also have a small effect in decreasing blood cholesterol in their own right because of their soluble fiber content. They can be eaten freely because they do not contribute to obesity and can enhance the variety of a healthy diet enormously. They may even protect against CVD in other ways, for example by providing antioxidants and folic acid.

Fiber. There is probably no point in deliberately advising individuals to consume high-fiber foods, particularly those rich in insoluble fiber. Wheat bran has no effect on blood cholesterol, and the so-called high-fiber diet has deterred many people from following a cholesterol-lowering diet.

Dietary cholesterol does not contribute greatly to blood cholesterol levels. It is probably wise to limit eggs to about three a week, but most patients can still enjoy avocado or shellfish when they get the chance. Foods are often labeled 'low in cholesterol'. This is unimportant. What is important is that they are 'low in saturated fat' if your patient is concerned with lowering blood cholesterol, and 'low in fat' if the patient is mainly trying to lose weight.

Carbohydrate. Refined carbohydrate, such as sugar in drinks and confectionery, should be avoided if the patient is trying to lose weight. The less-refined carbohydrate foods, such as bread, rice, pasta, beans and potatoes, have a much lower energy content than fat, and their consumption should be encouraged (in moderation for those trying to lose weight).

Coffee. There is probably no point in restricting coffee intake as a means of lowering blood cholesterol, because its effect is small.

Alcohol is not harmful to the heart in moderate amounts, and red wine, in moderate amounts, may reduce cardiovascular risk. However, in the obese, alcohol may be a major source of excess energy intake. In hyperlipidemia, particularly when associated with raised triglyceride levels, and in hypertension, it may be necessary to monitor a period of abstinence to assess the effects of alcohol.

Key points – dietary treatment

- Weight loss is the key strategy for the obese individual with dyslipidemia.
- Eating less works.
- Exercise is more helpful in maintaining weight loss than in achieving it.
- Alcohol is hypercaloric.

Key references

Durrington PN. Diet. In: *Hyperlipidaemia: Diagnosis and Management*, 3rd edn. London: Hodder Arnold, 2007:214–57.

Grundy SM. Dietary therapy of hyperlipidaemia. *Baillieres Clin Endocrinol Metab* 1987;1:667–98.

Haslam D, Wittert G. *Fast Facts: Obesity*. Oxford: Health Press Ltd, 2009.

Noakes M, Clifton P. Weight loss, diet composition and cardiovascular risk. *Curr Opin Lipidol* 2004;15: 31–5.

Vascular disease, whether coronary, cerebral or peripheral, is an absolute indication for intensive dietary and pharmacological therapy, as are genetic hyperlipoproteinemias (e.g. familial hypercholesterolemia [FH] and familial dysbetalipoproteinemia) and diabetes mellitus. For most other patients, the decision to treat and the target for therapy are based on the total risk of disease. Different schemes have been presented to incorporate the risk attributable to age, blood lipids and blood pressure, and the likelihood of a major clinical event calculated over, usually, a 10-year period. These are reviewed in Chapter 11.

Dietary modification is advocated either before lipid-lowering drugs are considered in lower-risk patients or at the same time as the initiation of lipid-lowering medication when the risk is higher. Unfortunately, diet alone is rarely more than partially successful, and the reality for most individuals is that medication is required to achieve major changes in plasma lipoprotein levels.

However impressive its safety record to date, lipid-lowering pharmacological therapy potentially carries some risk, which should never be overlooked. Moreover, the costs of therapy are substantial. They include not only the costs of the medication, but also all the associated costs, such as laboratory, medical and nursing resources. But the costs go even further. There is loss of time from work to attend clinics and there is often an increase in absenteeism in those labeled with diagnoses of chronic medical conditions. That said, in those who can benefit, pharmacological therapy is well justified.

Statins

Statins inhibit 3-hydroxy-3-methylglutaryl coenzyme A reductase, the physiologically rate-limiting enzyme for cholesterol biosynthesis. Their principal effect is to lower plasma low-density lipoprotein (LDL) (both LDL cholesterol and particle number), though modest increases in high-density lipoprotein (HDL) cholesterol and, depending on the agent and dose, variable decreases in plasma triglycerides also result. Postprandial remnant clearance may also be improved in some patients.

By altering the balance of cholesterol and cholesteryl ester within the hepatocyte, statins increase the removal of intermediate-density lipoprotein and LDL, and decrease the production of very-low-density lipoprotein (VLDL) and LDL. Although a number of non-lipoprotein effects have been reported, such as a decrease in C-reactive protein, the effects on the plasma lipoproteins – in particular the marked decrease in LDL – would appear to be the major mechanisms underlying clinical benefit.

There have been more than 20 statin trials with clinical events as outcomes. Most have involved randomizing patients to a trial statin and to placebo or usual care as a control group, whereas five trials have compared a less intensive statin regimen with a more intensive one. The overall findings are fascinating and have, in a short space of time, revolutionized our view of the management of dyslipidemia – international bodies advising on cardiovascular disease (CVD) prevention or evaluating statins for reimbursement by socialized healthcare systems have struggled to keep up with progress.

The trials establish that the risk of CVD (coronary heart disease [CHD] and stroke) is decreased by 21% for each 1 mmol/L (39 mg/dL) decrease in LDL cholesterol (Figure 10.1). CHD risk is decreased by 23% and stroke by 19% for each 1 mmol/L (39 mg/dL) decrease in LDL cholesterol. Another way of putting this is that CHD incidents decrease by around 1.25% for each 1% decrease in LDL cholesterol (Figure 10.2).

From meta-analyses of the statin trials, the following questions may be answered.

Is there a difference between primary and secondary prevention?
No. The relative decrease in CVD risk for a given decrease in LDL cholesterol is the same regardless of whether CHD or other atherosclerotic disease is already clinically evident. The absolute CVD risk determines how many new events will be prevented. The rate at which these are prevented is calculated by multiplying the absolute

CVD risk in a particular group of patients by the relative risk reduction

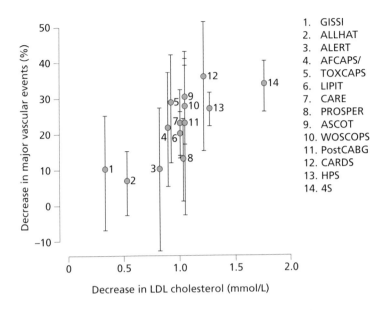

Figure 10.1 The percentage decrease in major vascular events (combined coronary heart disease and stroke) in actively treated patients compared with controls in 14 randomized trials, plotted as a function of the mean decrease in low-density lipoprotein (LDL) cholesterol concentrations compared with controls. The vertical lines show the 95% confidence intervals. Data from Baigent et al., 2005.

from statin treatment demonstrated in clinical trials. It is generally greatest in patients who already have CVD. However, the risk in primary prevention in some patients overlaps with that in secondary prevention. Absolute risk should determine who can benefit from statins, and these cannot logically be restricted to secondary prevention. Absolute risk is often expressed over the next 10 years, but this makes little sense in people whose life expectancy may be longer than this. Consequently, there is a move to consider lifetime risk (see later).

Does the pre-treatment lipid level matter? The statin-induced reduction in relative CVD risk is the same regardless of the pre-treatment LDL cholesterol, certainly between 2 mmol/L (80 mg/dL) and 5 mmol/L (200 mg/dL) or more. The implication of this is that the pre-treatment

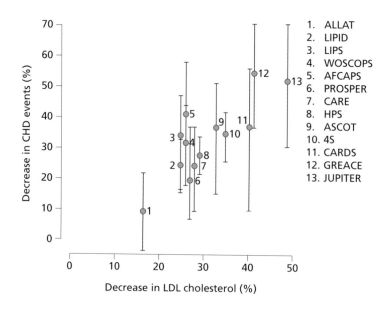

Figure 10.2 The percentage decrease in coronary heart disease as a function of the percentage decrease in low-density lipoprotein (LDL) cholesterol in actively treated, non-renal-transplant patients compared with controls in randomized statin trials lasting 3 years or more. The vertical lines show the 95% confidence intervals. Reference details for the data sources are provided at the end of this chapter.

LDL cholesterol level need not be high for a patient to benefit from statin treatment or, to put it another way, if a patient is at high CVD risk, then whatever his or her LDL cholesterol is, it is too high. This has led some to question whether it is necessary to measure lipid levels in high-risk patients if the maximum dose of a potent statin is to be given anyway, as is often the case, for example, immediately after acute myocardial infarction. Measuring lipid levels is important, however, to check compliance with treatment and to decide whether some adjunctive treatment is required in patients who have not achieved the recommended LDL cholesterol target (see Chapter 11).

In the statin trials the benefit from statins in terms of relative CVD risk reduction was also similar in people with high and low HDL cholesterol and in those with hypertriglyceridemia and normal triglyceride levels. Statin treatment is thus first-line treatment when HDL is low and/or triglycerides are raised, even though other drugs may increase HDL or lower triglyceride levels more effectively.

Does it matter what constitutes CVD risk? As long as the CVD risk is from atherosclerosis, the particular combination of risk factors does not affect the statin-induced reduction in risk. This is true of age (the strongest CVD risk factor), sex (the second strongest), diabetes, lipids, hypertension and smoking. Obviously absolute risk rises with age, so statin treatment prevents even more events in old people than in young people over a few years. But statin treatment should not be reserved for older people. Young people with genetic abnormalities such as FH clearly require therapy. More generally, for those with more than one major risk factor, more events will be prevented by early intervention than by waiting until some arbitrary absolute risk is achieved (Table 10.1).

Are statins safe? Randomized placebo-controlled trials have established that statins are generally safe. Although myalgia and minor increases in creatine kinase occur a little more commonly than with placebo, the incidence of rhabdomyolysis is less than 1 in 50 000 per person-year of treatment. Of course, aches and pains are part of everyday existence and many patients persuade themselves that they are experiencing

TABLE 10.1

Comparison of the number of coronary heart disease (CHD) deaths prevented by statin treatment to the age of 75 years in 1000 20-year-olds and 1000 70-year-olds, assuming statin treatment decreases risk by one-third.

Age (years)	Current annual CHD mortality	Average annual risk during rest of life	Decrease with statin therapy	Life expectancy (years)	Event-free life-years
20	1/1000	30/1000	10/1000	55	550/1000
70	60/1000	60/1000	20/1000	5	100/1000

statin-induced muscle symptoms. The clinician, at least, should appreciate that in the randomized trials almost as many patients receiving placebo-treatment believed they had statin-induced myalgia. Too frequently this important group of drugs is denied to patients at high CVD risk in the mistaken belief that they are statin intolerant. Generally, all that is required is careful explanation and perhaps a change to a different statin. Certainly minor asymptomatic increases in creatine kinase of up to 1000 IU/L (and sometimes higher if the patient has an occupation or leisure pursuit requiring physical exertion) are not a reason to discontinue statin treatment. Remember too that normal reference ranges for creatine kinase are higher in people of African ancestry. Caution should be exercised if a patient is receiving medication known to interact with statins, such as bezafibrate, fenofibrate, ciprofibrate, amiodarone, diltiazem, verapamil or ciclosporin. The combination of certain drugs with statins should be avoided altogether. These include macrolide antibiotics, imidazole and triazole antifungals (stop the statin if these are essential), and gemfibrozil. Patients with untreated hypothyroidism are also at increased risk of myositis, but not when established on adequate thyroxine treatment.

Statin-induced hepatic dysfunction is also rare in randomized clinical trials. Clinicians who insist on measuring γ-glutamyl transpeptidase and hepatic transaminases will find that these fluctuate and, indeed, because non-alcohol hepatic steatohepatitis (NASH) is more common in hyperlipidemia, abnormal levels will be encountered, giving the impression that they have increased with statin treatment. Again, care should be taken to avoid stopping statin treatment unnecessarily under such circumstances. On the other hand, of course, it is important to ensure that there is no underlying primary liver disease other than NASH or that one of the other drugs the patient is receiving is not proving hepatotoxic.

Are statins safe in renal disease? Statins are generally safe in renal disease and after renal transplantation, though special care needs to be taken to avoid drug interactions. Clinical trial evidence of CVD benefit in advanced renal disease is lacking, but patients with creatinine levels up to 200 µmol/L benefit and do not experience any statin-induced deterioration in glomerular function or in proteinuria.

How low should the target LDL cholesterol be? Conceptually, the answer is simple: the lower the LDL cholesterol, the lower the risk. In practice, however, the authorities that guide practice have produced a series of targets depending on the indication for treatment. These different indications are outlined in detail in Chapter 11. The targets for secondary prevention are sometimes lower than for primary prevention. In the UK, the Joint British Societies 2 (JBS2) target for statin treatment for secondary prevention is LDL cholesterol below 2 mmol/L (80 mg/dL). In the USA, the target recommended by ATPIII for secondary prevention is LDL cholesterol below 2.6 mmol/L (100 mg/dL) with the option of aiming for less than 1.8 mmol/L (70 mg/dL) for very-high-risk subjects.

In the USA, two LDL cholesterol targets for primary prevention of 3.3 and 4.0 mmol/L (130 and 160 mg/dL) have been adopted depending on the precise level of risk. In the UK, the definition of CVD risk in primary prevention also includes the risk of developing angina or cerebrovascular disease. For non-diabetic patients, no primary prevention statin target for LDL cholesterol is recommended by the National Institute for Health and Clinical Excellence (NICE), but it has adopted the 2.0 mmol/L (80 mg/dL) target proposed by the JBS2 guidelines for diabetes and secondary prevention. The NICE policy of using simvastatin, 40 mg daily, as the sole first-line treatment in primary prevention seems inappropriate in patients whose LDL cholesterol is too high to achieve even the Department of Health general practice audit target of 3 mmol/L (120 mg/dL) or its equivalent total cholesterol of 5 mmol/L (200 mg/dL) or less without the prescription of a more potent statin.

The evidence for lowering LDL cholesterol below 1.8 or 2.0 mmol/L (70 or 80 mg/dL) in diabetes comes from the Collaborative Atorvastatin Diabetes Study (CARDS), the primary prevention trial of atorvastatin, 10 mg daily, versus placebo in type 2 diabetes. The mean pre-treatment LDL cholesterol was 3 mmol/L (120 mg/dL) and the typical patient receiving active treatment in the trial achieved LDL cholesterol levels below 2 mmol/L (80 mg/dL); this led to a 37% decrease in CVD events. Benefit was not attenuated in those whose pre-treatment LDL cholesterol was below 3 mmol/L (< 120 mg/dL) compared with those in whom it was higher. In the Medical Research Council/British Heart Foundation Heart Protection Study (HPS), in which there was a large diabetic cohort without previous vascular disease, pre-treatment LDL cholesterol was similar to that in CARDS. Although, overall, simvastatin, 40 mg daily, was less effective than atorvastatin, 10 mg daily, the patients in HPS with the lower pre-treatment LDL cholesterol but whose levels on treatment were below 2 mmol/L achieved the same decrease in relative CVD risk as those with a similar decrease in LDL cholesterol from higher pre-treatment levels. The results of the Cholesterol Treatment Trialists (CTT) meta-analysis are quite clear: the greater the LDL cholesterol decrease, the greater the decrease in CVD risk.

So why not decrease LDL cholesterol from whatever its pre-treatment value to less than 2.0 or 1.8 mmol/L (80 mg/dL or 70 mg/dL)? For an LDL cholesterol level of 4 mmol/L (160 mg/dL), a decrease of 2 mmol/L (80 mg/dL) would be expected to achieve a 42% decrease in CVD events rather than only the 21% which would result from a 1 mmol/L (40 mg/dL) decrease to 3 mmol/L (120 mg/dL). This proposition has been shown to work well in patients who already have CHD in trials in which more intensive statin treatment regimens have been compared with less intensive ones. A meta-analysis has shown that an additional decrease in LDL cholesterol to levels of, on average, 1.9 mmol/L (75 mg/dL) with intensive statin treatment, rather than the 2.6 mmol/L (101 mg/dL) achieved with standard doses, produces a further 16% decrease in CVD risk – slightly more than would be predicted from the CTT meta-analysis.

It may be difficult to get some patients with particularly high pre-treatment LDL cholesterol to target even with high doses of the more potent statins combined with other cholesterol-lowering medication. Some comfort can be derived from the possibility that by decreasing LDL cholesterol from, say, 6 mmol/L to 3 mmol/L, a 63% decrease in CVD risk may have been achieved, even if the additional 21% decrease possible by reducing LDL cholesterol to 2 mmol/L cannot be realized.

In our view, therefore, the evidence for aiming for LDL cholesterol levels below 1.8 or 2.0 mmol/L (70 or 80 mg/dL) is overwhelming. Our only reservation is that we would prefer the LDL treatment target to be couched in terms of apoB, the indicator of LDL particle concentration, because it is surprising how much LDL can still be circulating in patients who have achieved an LDL cholesterol level of 1.8 mmol/L (70 mg/dL), particularly in those with diabetes or hypertriglyceridemia in whom cholesterol-depleted LDL is prevalent. Statins lower LDL cholesterol substantially more than they lower apoB. The Canadian Cardiovascular Society has recommended an apoB target of less than 85 mg/dL. As displayed in Table 10.2, the recent Consensus Statements of the American Diabetes Association (ADA) and the American College of Cardiology (ACC) recommend: 1) that apoB is the best measure of the adequacy of LDL lowering therapy and 2) that high-risk patients be treated to a level of less than 90 mg/dL whereas very-high-risk patients should be treated to a level of less than 80 mg/dL.

How rapidly do statins reduce CVD risk? CVD risk declines rapidly on the introduction of statin therapy (Figure 10.3). It is statistically significant after 1 year and within 2 years the full decrease in relative CVD risk is achieved. Relative CVD is the ratio between the number of events in patients treated with statins and in those receiving a placebo. So the fact that the full relative risk reduction is achieved early on does not mean that the statin benefit is complete by 2 years because, of

TABLE 10.2

ADA and ACC targets for LDL lowering strategies

	High-risk patients	Very-high-risk patients
ApoB*	< 90 mg/dL	< 80 mg/dL
LDL-C	< 100 mg/dL	< 70 mg/dL
	(2.5 mmol/L)	(1.8 mmol/L)

*Achieving the apoB target should be the primary aim. As apoB measurement is not currently available to many clinicians, a low-density lipoprotein cholesterol (LDL-C) target is also identified.

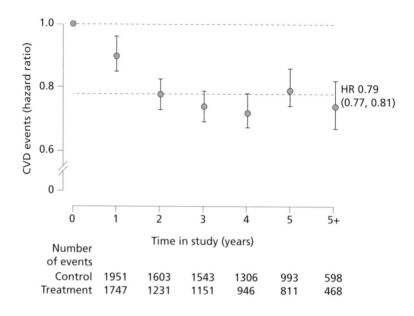

Figure 10.3 The ratio of the rate of cardiovascular disease (CVD) events in patients receiving active treatment compared with controls (hazard ratio, HR) for each 1 mmol/L (40 mg/dL) difference in LDL cholesterol in 14 randomized statin trials, plotted against the duration of treatment in the study. The vertical lines show the 95% confidence intervals. A statistically significant decrease in HR was evident at 1 year; by 2 years the relative difference in risk that was to persist throughout the trial had been achieved. Data from Baigent et al., 2005.

course, the CVD event rate in the placebo group increases exponentially and so, therefore, does the number of events prevented by the statin. Hence, the additional benefit of longer treatment (Table 10.1).

Are statins cost effective? Yes. Unfortunately, cost effectiveness is not well understood. Generally, if an intervention provides one quality-adjusted life year (QALY) at a cost under £30 000 ($58 000), it is considered cost effective. Even at levels of risk greatly below those currently recommended in the UK, the rest of Europe and the USA, statins, particularly simvastatin, would be judged cost effective. The reason many countries have limited the use of statins to patients whose

10-year CVD risk is 20% or more is because there are so many people at this high level of risk that the *total* cost of statin treatment would be extremely high. Doctors and nurses need to be cautious in their explanation as to why they are not prescribing a statin to individuals whose risk is below, but close to, 20% over 10 years. Many might be deeply resentful to learn they might avoid a CVD event for little more than $4–6 or £2–3 per month. This dilemma was the main motivation for the introduction in England and Wales of over-the-counter simvastatin at the discretion of the pharmacist, though this is only available at a dose of 10 mg and at a higher cost to the consumer than the cost of the equivalent dose to the National Health Service. With examples like this, it is not hard to see why clinical guidelines everywhere are in a state of flux, though fortunately they are evolving slowly in more logical directions.

Other lipid-lowering drugs

Fibrates. The mechanism of action of fibrates involves stimulation of the peroxisome proliferator-activated receptor α. This leads to decreased triglyceride production by the liver and improved triglyceride clearance by peripheral tissues. The most important clinical effects are a marked reduction in serum triglycerides and an increase in HDL cholesterol. Depending on the agent and the type of hyperlipidemia, LDL cholesterol and apoB levels may be reduced, but not usually by more than 10–20%. Postprandial triglyceride clearance is also improved after fibrate therapy.

Overall, randomized clinical trials of fibrate drugs have not produced clear evidence of a substantial positive effect on CHD risk. The strongest evidence is for gemfibrozil in secondary prevention in the Veterans Affairs High-density Lipoprotein Cholesterol Intervention Trial (VA-HIT). On the other hand, the risk of severe muscle injury, either on its own or in combination therapy with statin, is highest with gemfibrozil. The Fenofibrate Intervention and Event Lowering in Diabetes (FIELD) trial, which tested fenofibrate, did not achieve its primary endpoint nor did the Action to Control Cardiovascular Risk in Diabetes (ACCORD) trial, which tested fenofibrate plus statin against statin. At this point, there is no significant evidence base on which to recommend fibrate therapy to reduce cardiovascular events.

So what can we conclude about fibrates? Fibrates are certainly the pharmacological agents of choice in individuals who, by virtue of markedly elevated triglyceride levels, are at risk of pancreatitis. Normalization of plasma lipids also commonly occurs in patients with familial dysbetalipoproteinemia. In other patients with vascular disease, lack of trial data demonstrating clinical efficacy of fibrates means statin treatment should be the first-line therapy. It is possible that in subgroups such as those with metabolic syndrome with or without diabetes, fibrates may bring particular benefit, given the characteristic lipid profile of hypertriglyceridemia, low HDL cholesterol and small, dense LDL, but against a background of statin treatment this awaits confirmation. Although the strongest current evidence is for gemfibrozil in secondary prevention, gemfibrozil is the most strongly contraindicated member of this class of drugs in combination with a statin, because of the high risk of myositis. Gemfibrozil can really only be considered in patients who are not receiving any statin treatment, having proven intolerant of the whole gamut of such drugs.

Side effects with fibrates are generally mild. Headache, gastrointestinal upset, rashes and pruritus have been reported. Mild elevations of hepatic and muscle enzymes may occur. Bile lithogenicity is probably increased, at least in the early stages of treatment. Fibrates should be avoided in patients known to have gallstones, though only clofibrate has been shown in clinical trials to increase the incidence of clinically significant cholelithiasis.

Fibrates may interact significantly with anticoagulants such as warfarin, and great care should be exercised in their introduction in patients receiving such therapy. Their use should be avoided in patients with renal disease (bezafibrate, in particular, raises creatinine levels) and they may cause a paradoxical rise in cholesterol in patients with cholestatic liver disease, in whom they are contraindicated.

Ezetimibe inhibits cholesterol absorption, probably by downregulating Niemann–Pick C1 Like 1 protein in the brush border of enterocytes. Reduced delivery of cholesterol to the liver results in lower LDL levels in plasma. Ezetimibe is administered once a day at a single dose of 10 mg. In patients intolerant to statins, monotherapy with ezetimibe will lower LDL cholesterol and apoB by about 20%. The more common usage is in combination with statins. This allows lower doses of statins to be used so that side effects can be minimized or, if higher doses of more potent statins are used, LDL can be lowered even further. There are as yet no trial data to confirm that ezetimibe decreases CVD risk.

To date, there has been little evidence of ezetimibe hepatoxicity, and drug interactions characteristic of bile-acid resins have not been reported. Ciclosporin significantly alters the plasma kinetics of ezetimibe, but the as yet limited clinical data on ezetimibe combined with fibrates are encouraging. With careful monitoring, ezetimibe in combination with gemfibrozil may, therefore, be considered for secondary prevention in patients with mixed hyperlipidemia who are intolerant of statins.

Bile-acid resins. These are non-absorbable anion-exchange resins that bind bile salts, so preventing their reabsorption from the terminal ileum. The resulting depletion in the bile-acid pool leads to greater breakdown of cholesterol to form bile acids. In turn, this leads to upregulation of LDL receptors to maintain the cholesterol pool within the liver, and lowering of LDL levels, typically by 10–20% (more in compliant patients). Plasma triglyceride levels, however, may increase substantially, particularly in those with already elevated levels.

The major indication for these agents is in combination with a statin in patients with very high LDL levels. There may be an increased likelihood of gallstone development with bile-acid sequestrants, though this may be lower in patients already receiving statins. Bile-acid sequestrants can decrease serum folate levels, and folate supplementation should be considered in vulnerable groups, such as women who may become pregnant and children. In the Lipid Research Clinics Trial, colestyramine decreased CHD incidence, and both colestyramine and colestipol have been used alone or in combination with other drugs in successful coronary angiographic regression trials. Evidence that they significantly decrease all-cause mortality is not available, however, and it is unlikely that further trials will be undertaken to test this. Constipation, bloating and heartburn are common side effects with colestyramine and colestipol, limiting their usefulness. Colesevelam, a newer bile-acid-sequestrating agent in tablet form (as opposed to colestyramine and colestipol, which are powders that must be soaked in water or fruit juice) is reportedly better tolerated, despite dosages of 1875 mg (three tablets) twice daily with meals or 3750 mg (six tablets) once daily with a meal.

Nicotinic acid is a B vitamin that, in pharmacological doses (up to 7 g daily), markedly reduces VLDL and LDL and substantially increases HDL. It alone among the hypolipidemic agents may reduce lipoprotein (a). Its mechanism of action is not certain, but involves reducing VLDL secretion by the liver, perhaps in response to reduced fatty acid release by adipocytes.

The advantages of nicotinic acid are that it improves the whole lipoprotein profile, and its cost is low. Opinions are divided about whether the dose should be taken all at once with the evening meal, allowing flushing (see below) to be endured in the privacy of one's own home, or whether it should be taken in divided doses to try to minimize side effects. In either case, it is customary to begin with 50 mg daily, working up to a dose of 3000 mg or above. The dose should be taken at the end of a meal with a small dose of aspirin at the beginning. Lipoprotein levels should be assessed 1 month later.

Flushing, which is prostaglandin mediated, is virtually universal. Although flushing can be partially ameliorated by aspirin, a more specific blocker of the prostaglandin receptor involved in nicotinic acid-induced flushing, laropiprant, is currently undergoing clinical trials. Because of the flushing, earlier clinical trials – though supportive of the hypothesis that nicotinic acid decreases CHD risk, particularly in metabolic syndrome – cannot be regarded as double- or even single-blinded. More serious side effects include gastritis and peptic ulcer exacerbation, hepatitis, gout and hyperglycemia. Significant interaction with statins can occur to produce rhabdomyolysis and renal failure.

Because of its attractive effect on the lipoprotein profile, numerous attempts have been made to produce analogs or slow-release preparations of nicotinic acid that overcome the flushing problems. In many cases, these have simply made the flushing reaction unpredictable. Acipimox does appear to induce less flushing, but though it retains the triglyceride-lowering action of its parent nicotinic acid, it is much less effective at lowering serum cholesterol. Niaspan is also designed to minimize flushing; in addition to lowering cholesterol and triglycerides, it can increase HDL cholesterol effectively.

Strategies to achieve maximal LDL-lowering

Many patients with LDL cholesterol levels of 3–4 mmol/L (120–160 mg/dL) or below can achieve LDL cholesterol levels below 1.80–2.0 mmol/L (70–80 mg/dL) with: simvastatin, 40 mg daily; atorvastatin, 10 mg daily; or rosuvastatin, 5 mg daily. Patients with higher LDL cholesterol levels require higher doses of atorvastatin or rosuvastatin to achieve target LDL cholesterol or, even better, apoB. Doubling the dose of a statin produces, on average, a further 6% decrease in LDL cholesterol. Typical reductions in LDL cholesterol with different statins in their approved dose ranges are shown in Figure 10.4. An alternative

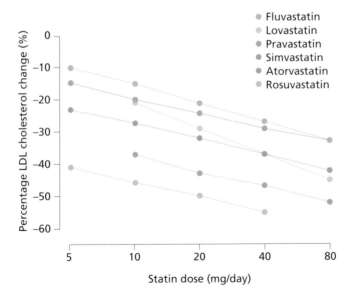

Figure 10.4 Overview of reported LDL-cholesterol-lowering effect of different statins in their approved dose ranges. The data are from Law MR et al. *BMJ* 2003;326:1423–7 and Wlodarczyk J et al. *Am J Cardiol* 2008;102:1654–62.

strategy is to use a statin plus either ezetimibe or bile-acid resins. Ezetimibe appears to be better tolerated than the bile-acid resins. Such combinations allow lower doses of statins to be used and the frequency of low-grade, statin-induced muscle ache to be reduced. On the other hand, two drugs must be used and the cost should be considered. A single pill containing simvastatin and ezetimibe is available. Some patients, such as those with FH, will require maximum doses of statin and a second agent such as ezetimibe, and occasionally a bile-acid sequestrant or nicotinic acid, to approach target levels.

Combination strategies to lower LDL, reduce small, dense LDL and increase HDL. A statin plus a fibrate can be used. The combination does increase the risk of myositis, and patients, who should be those likely to concord with management (taking medicines as prescribed and keeping follow-up appointments), must be carefully monitored. Gemfibrozil, for which there is most evidence for benefit as monotherapy, should not be used for this purpose. The principal effects of the statin will be to reduce apoB and LDL cholesterol. Some decrease in small, dense LDL will also occur, but particularly in combined hyperlipidemia, smaller, denser LDL particles will persist. A fibrate will lower triglycerides further and this will produce a shift from small, denser LDL particles to larger, more buoyant LDL particles. Given the current uncertainty about the role of fibrates, evidence that combination with statin therapy increases clinical benefit would be welcome, but unfortunately is not available.

The combination of a statin and purified omega-3 fatty acids should also be considered, particularly as the risk of myositis is not increased and a favorable effect of purified omega-3 fatty acids on CHD risk has been reported against a background of statin therapy (GISSI and JELIS). These effects were, however, reported with lower doses than the 4 g daily dose which is often required to lower triglycerides by an amount comparable with that achieved with a fibrate.

Alternatively, a statin plus nicotinic acid can be prescribed. The combination of simvastatin and nicotinic acid has been tested in the HDL–Atherosclerosis Treatment Study (HATS) in individuals with coronary disease, LDL cholesterol at or below 3.62 mmol/L (145 mg/dL) and low HDL cholesterol. The combination lowered LDL cholesterol by

42%, increased HDL cholesterol by 26% and HDL2 by 65%, reduced clinical events and induced angiographic regression of coronary disease; antioxidant vitamins appeared to reduce the degree of benefit.

At the moment, there are no therapies clinically proven to decrease CVD risk by raising HDL. Thus, in patients with low HDL, lowering LDL cholesterol or apoB to an appropriately low target is the most evidence-based approach.

Key points – drug treatment

- Statins reduce coronary heart disease and cerebrovascular disease events by about one-fifth, in both primary and secondary prevention, for each 1 mmol/L (40 mg/dL) decrease in low-density lipoprotein (LDL) cholesterol.
- Evidence of clinical benefit is clear for statins, but equivocal for fibrates.
- Much controversy remains as to the targets of statin therapy. Our view of the evidence is that lower is better, and that therapy guided by the apoB level may be even more effective than that guided by LDL cholesterol level.
- The apoB/apoAI ratio is the best summary index of the risk of vascular disease and may well turn out to be the best summary index of the adequacy of lipid-lowering therapy (see chapter 12).

Key references

Armitage J. The safety of statins in clinical practice. *Lancet* 2007;370: 1781–90.

Athyros VG, Papageorgiou AA, Mercouris BR et al. Treatment with atorvastatin to the National Cholesterol Education Program goal versus 'usual' care in secondary coronary heart disease prevention. The GREek Atorvastatin and Coronary-heart-disease Evaluation (GREACE) study. *Curr Med Res Opin* 2002;18:220–8.

Baigent C, Keech A, Kearney PM et al.; Cholesterol Treatment Trialists' (CTT) Collaborators. Efficacy and safety of cholesterol-lowering treatment: prospective meta-analysis of data from 90,056 participants in 14 randomised trials of statins. *Lancet* 2005;366:1267–78.

Bays H, Jones PH. Colesevelam hydrochloride: reducing atherosclerotic coronary heart disease risk factors. *Vasc Health Risk Manag* 2007;3:733–42.

Birjmohun RS, Hutten BA, Kastelein JJ, Stroes ES. Efficacy and safety of high-density lipoprotein cholesterol-increasing compounds. A meta-analysis of randomized controlled trials. *J Am Coll Cardiol* 2005;45:185–97.

Brunzell JD, Davidson M, Furberg CD et al. Lipoprotein management in patients with cardiometabolic risk: consensus statement from the American Diabetes Association and the American College of Cardiology Foundation. *Diabetes Care* 2008;31:811–22.

Canner PL, Furberg CD, McGovern ME. Benefits of niacin in patients with versus without the metabolic syndrome and healed myocardial infarction (from the Coronary Drug Project). *Am J Cardiol* 2006;97:477–9.

Cannon CP, Steinberg BA, Murphy SA et al. Meta-analysis of cardiovascular outcomes trials comparing intensive versus moderate statin therapy. *J Am Coll Cardiol* 2006;48:438–45.

Colhoun HM, Betteridge DJ, Durrington PN et al. Primary prevention of cardiovascular disease with atorvastatin in type 2 diabetes in the Collaborative Atorvastatin Diabetes Study (CARDS): multicentre randomised placebo-controlled trial. *Lancet* 2004;364:685–96.

Collins R, Armitage J, Parish S et al.; Heart Protection Study Collaborative Group. MRC/BHF Heart Protection Study of cholesterol-lowering with simvastatin in 5963 people with diabetes: a randomised placebo-controlled trial. *Lancet* 2003;361: 2005–16.

Collins R, Armitage J, Parish S et al.; Heart Protection Study Collaborative Group. Effects of cholesterol-lowering with simvastatin on stroke and other major vascular events in 20,536 people with cerebrovascular disease or other high-risk conditions. *Lancet* 2004;363:757–67.

Contois JH, McConnell JP, Sethi AA et al.; AACC Lipoproteins and Vascular Diseases Division Working Group on Best Practices. Apolipoprotein B and cardiovascular disease risk: position statement from the AACC Lipoproteins and Vascular Diseases Division Working Group on Best Practices. *Clin Chem* 2009;55:407–19.

Durrington PN, Bhatnagar D, Mackness MI et al. An omega-3 polyunsaturated fatty acid concentrate administered for one year decreased triglycerides in simvastatin treated patients with coronary heart disease and persisting hypertriglyceridaemia. *Heart* 2001; 85:544–8.

Frick MH, Elo H, Haapa K et al. Helsinki Heart Study: primary-prevention trial with gemfibrozil in middle-aged men with dyslipidemia. Safety of treatment, changes in risk factors, and incidence of coronary heart disease. *N Engl J Med* 1987; 317:1237–45.

Gissi-HF Investigators: Tavazzi L, Maggioni AP, Marchioli R et al. Effect of rosvastatin in patients with chronic heart failure (the GISSI-HF trial): a randomised, double-blind, placebo-controlled trial. *Lancet* 2008;372:1231–9.

GISSI-Prevenzione Investigators. Dietary supplementation with n-3 polyunsaturated fatty acids and vitamin E after myocardial infarction: results of the GISSI-Prevenzione trial. *Lancet* 1999;354: 447–55.

Gotto AM, Farmer JA. Drug insight: the role of statins in combination with ezetimibe to lower LDL cholesterol. *Nat Clin Pract Cardiovasc Med* 2006;3:664–72.

Heart Protection Study Collaborative Group. MRC/BHF Heart Protection Study of cholesterol lowering with simvastatin in 20,536 high-risk individuals: a randomised placebo-controlled trial. *Lancet* 2002;360:7–22.

Keech A, Simes RJ, Barter P et al.; FIELD study investigators. Effects of long-term fenofibrate therapy on cardiovascular events in 9795 people with type 2 diabetes mellitus (the FIELD study): randomised controlled trial. *Lancet* 2005;366:1849–61.

Law MR, Wald NJ, Rudnicka AR. Quantifying effect of statins on low density lipoprotein cholesterol, ischaemic heart disease, and stroke: systematic review and meta-analysis. *BMJ* 2003;326:1423–7.

Marchioli R, Barzi F, Bomba E et al. Early protection against sudden death by n-3 polyunsaturated fatty acids after myocardial infarction. Time course analysis of the results of the Gruppo Italiano per lo Studio della Sopravvivenza nell'Infarto Miocardico (GISSI) – Prevenzione. *Circulation* 2002;105:1897–903.

National Institute for Health and Clinical Excellence. Statins for the prevention of cardiovascular events. *Technology Appraisal* 94. London: National Institute for Health and Clinical Excellence, 2006.

Oliver MF, Heady JA, Morris JN et al. A co-operative trial in the primary prevention of ischaemic heart disease using clofibrate: a report from the Committee of Principal Investigators. *Br Heart J* 1978;40:106–18.

Paolini JF, Mitchel YB, Reyes R et al. Effects of laropiprant on nicotinic acid-induced flushing in patients with dyslipidemia. *Am J Cardiol* 2008;101:625–30.

Ridker PM, Danielson E, Fonseca FA et al. Rosuvastatin to prevent vascular events in men and women with elevated C-reactive protein. *N Engl J Med* 2008;359:2195–207.

Roeters van Lennep JE, Westerveld HT, Roeters van Lennep HWO et al. Apolipoprotein concentrations during treatment and recurrent coronary artery disease events. *Arterioscler Thromb Vasc Biol* 2000;20:2408–13.

Rubins HB, Rubins SJ, Collins D et al. Gemfibrozil for the secondary prevention of coronary heart disease in men with low levels of high-density lipoprotein cholesterol. *N Engl J Med* 1999;341:410–18.

Scandinavian Simvastatin Survival Study Group. Randomised trial of cholesterol lowering in 4444 patients with coronary heart disease; the Scandinavian Survival Study. *Lancet* 1994;344:1383–9.

Smilde TJ, van Wissen S, Wollersheim H et al. Effect of aggressive versus conventional lipid lowering on atherosclerosis progression in familial hypercholesterolemia (ASAP): a prospective, randomised, double-blind trial. *Lancet* 2001;357:577–81.

Study of the Effectiveness of Additional Reductions in Cholesterol and Homocysteine (SEARCH). Information and results, when released, available at www.searchinfo.org

The ACCORD Study Group. Effects of combination lipid therapy in type 2 diabetes mellitus. *N Engl J Med* 2010 Mar 14. doi:10.1056/NEJMoa1001282.

The Lipid Research Clinics Program. The Lipid Research Clinics Coronary Primary Prevention Trial. Results I: Reduction in incidence of coronary heart disease. *JAMA* 1984;251: 351–64.

Yokoyama M, Origasa H, Matsuzaki M et al.; Japan EPA lipid intervention study (JELIS) Investigators. Effects of eicosapentaenoic acid on major coronary events in hyper-cholesterolaemic patients (JELIS): a randomised open-label, blinded end-point analysis. *Lancet* 2007:369: 1090–8.

Yusuf S, Hawken S, Ounpuu S et al.; INTERHEART Study Investigators. Effect of potentially modifiable risk factors associated with myocardial infarction in 52 countries (the INTERHEART study): case–control study. *Lancet* 2004;364:937–52.

Physicians now have an unparalleled opportunity to prevent vascular disease – but only if we act. We divide prevention strategies into those that apply to everyone and those that are necessary for selected groups. A healthy diet – a diet that is energy-neutral for the patient who is not obese and energy-negative for one who is, and that is not fatty-acid excessive – is the most neglected but powerful act of prevention. Promoting exercise is wonderful not only for health, but also for self-esteem. Helping patients to stop smoking is critical. These are the fundamentals to prevent vascular disease, and they apply to everyone, but unfortunately these objectives are easier to list than to implement.

However, there are also substantial numbers at high individual risk who need to be considered for pharmacological as well as dietary therapy. In almost all instances, this will mean statin therapy. Because vascular disease is so common and because pharmacological therapy remains expensive, certainly in the aggregate, deciding where to draw the line has major cost implications for any society. Medical experts have accepted this argument and have drawn up protocols to determine whether pharmacological therapy is justified. It is a fair question whether we can act both for society and our patients at the same time.

Clinical evidence of disease

There are three indications for pharmacological therapy based on clinical evidence of disease.

- Objective evidence of vascular disease. This includes any evidence of coronary, cerebrovascular or peripheral vascular disease. In addition to symptoms, electrocardiographic and angiographic evidence, this would include, in our judgment, ultrasound evidence of disease in the extracranial cerebral or peripheral vessels.
- The second absolute clinical indication is diabetes, either type 1 or type 2. The age at which hypolipidemic therapy should start remains unclear – the presence of additional risk factors such as nephropathy,

hypertension, marked dyslipidemia (Table 11.1) may militate in favor of treatment in a patient as young as 18 years of age.

- The third clinical indication is the presence of severe hyperlipidemia such as occurs in familial hypercholesterolemia (FH) (see Chapter 3), familial dysbetalipoproteinemia (see Chapter 6) and hypertriglyceridemia substantial enough to cause acute pancreatitis (see Chapter 5). Even though not linked to a specific metabolic cause, marked hypercholesterolemia or a very high serum total to HDL cholesterol ratio regardless of total cardiovascular disease (CVD) risk is often also accepted as an indication for therapy (see later).

Risk assessment

The importance of identifying asymptomatic individuals who will develop early and accelerated vascular disease has led to the development of numerous guidelines around the world. From this complex process, a consensus is gradually starting to emerge. The recent ATPIII guidelines base the decision to treat on overall risk rather than just the level of cholesterol. In this regard, the American approach now resembles that previously taken in Europe. Nevertheless, important differences remain between the American and European approaches summarized below.

The ATPIII approach is summarized in Figure 11.1. For those with two or more risk factors, risk should be calculated from the Framingham tables (Tables 11.1 and 11.2). The full ATPIII report was published in December 2002. An amended set of recommendations appeared in July 2004 based on a series of clinical trials completed in the intervening period. The most important of these was the HPS, which demonstrated that high-risk individuals with low-density lipoprotein (LDL) cholesterol below 2.5 mmol/L (100 mg/dL) – that is, at a level considered to be already at target – received similar proportionate benefit from statin therapy as those with values above this level. Accordingly, the amended recommendations provide an optional target value for LDL cholesterol of below 1.80 mmol/L (70 mg/dL) for a new category of very-high-risk individuals (those with a combination of risk factors such as diabetes and coronary disease). Additionally, those at intermediate risk have an optional LDL cholesterol target of below 2.5 mmol/L (100 mg/dL).

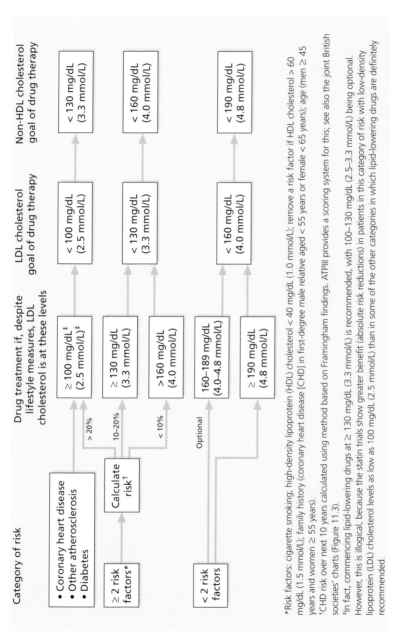

Figure 11.1 Synopsis of the third report of the National Cholesterol Education Program (NCEP) expert panel on detection, evaluation and treatment of high blood cholesterol in adults (Adult Treatment Panel III).

TABLE 11.1

Method of estimating 10-year risk of coronary heart disease for men (Framingham point scores) provided in ATPIII*

Age (years)	Points
20–34	–9
35–39	–4
40–44	0
45–49	3
50–54	6
55–59	8
60–64	10
65–69	11
70–74	12
75–79	13

Total cholesterol (mg/dL)	Points				
	Age 20–39 years	Age 40–49 years	Age 50–59 years	Age 60–69 years	Age 70–79 years
< 160	0	0	0	0	0
160–199	4	3	2	1	0
200–239	7	5	3	1	0
240–279	9	6	4	2	1
≥ 280	11	8	5	3	1

Smoking	Points				
	Age 20–39 years	Age 40–49 years	Age 50–59 years	Age 60–69 years	Age 70–79 years
Non-smoker	0	0	0	0	0
Smoker	8	5	3	1	1

TABLE 11.1 (CONTINUED)

HDL (mg/dL)	Points
≥ 60	−1
50–59	0
40–49	1
< 40	2

Systolic BP (mmHg)	If untreated	If treated
< 120	0	0
120–129	1	3
130–139	2	4
140–159	3	5
≥ 160	4	6

Point total	10-year risk (%)
< 9	< 1
9	1
10	1
11	1
12	1
13	2
14	2
15	3
16	4
17	5
18	6
19	8
20	11
21	14
22	17
23	22
24	27
≥ 25	≥ 30

*Third report of the National Cholesterol Education Program (NCEP) expert panel on the detection, evaluation and treatment of high blood cholesterol in adults (Adult Treatment Panel III), 2001.

TABLE 11.2

Method of estimating 10-year risk of coronary heart disease for women (Framingham point scores) provided in ATPIII*

Age (years)	Points
20–34	–7
35–39	–3
40–44	0
45–49	3
50–54	6
55–59	8
60–64	10
65–69	12
70–74	14
75–79	16

Total cholesterol (mg/dL)	Points				
	Age 20–39 years	Age 40–49 years	Age 50–59 years	Age 60–69 years	Age 70–79 years
< 160	0	0	0	0	0
160–199	4	3	2	1	1
200–239	8	6	4	2	1
240–279	11	8	5	3	2
≥ 280	13	10	7	4	2

Smoking	Points				
	Age 20–39 years	Age 40–49 years	Age 50–59 years	Age 60–69 years	Age 70–79 years
Non-smoker	0	0	0	0	0
Smoker	9	7	4	2	1

TABLE 11.2 (CONTINUED)

HDL (mg/dL)	Points
≥ 60	−1
50–59	0
40–49	1
< 40	2

Systolic BP (mmHg)	If untreated	If treated
< 120	0	0
120–129	0	1
130–139	1	2
140–159	1	2
≥ 160	2	3

Point total	10-year risk (%)
< 0	< 1
0	1
1	1
2	1
3	1
4	1
5	2
6	2
7	3
8	4
9	5
10	6
11	8
12	10
13	12
14	16
15	20
16	25
≥ 17	≥ 30

*Third report of the National Cholesterol Education Program (NCEP) expert panel on the detection, evaluation and treatment of high blood cholesterol in adults (Adult Treatment Panel III), 2001.

This is a more comprehensive approach, and we agree with this change in direction. However, there are a number of limitations.

- The multiple groups and targets will almost certainly be confusing for practitioners.
- Risk from lipids is calculated on the basis of total and HDL cholesterol, whereas the targets for therapy are levels of LDL cholesterol.
- The risk estimates are not valid for patients with FH, familial dysbetalipoproteinemia, diabetes or renal disease. These patients must be treated rigorously at whatever age they present.
- Hypertriglyceridemia, which is an independent risk factor for CHD (see Chapter 5), remains a problem because it is not included as such in the ATPIII guidelines. As we have noted, hypertriglyceridemia is common in coronary patients. ATPIII does acknowledge the issue by producing a definition of the metabolic syndrome. For these patients, it is suggested that risk and adequacy of therapy be gauged by non-HDL cholesterol, creating yet another number to remember and monitor. The apoB concentration, a measure of the number of LDL particles present, is available from some laboratories. The Canadian recommendations for the management of dyslipidemia and the prevention of CVD, while in many respects similar to ATPIII, include apoB exceeding 120 mg/dL together with serum triglycerides exceeding 1.5 mmol/L (135 mg/dL) as an indicator of high risk. They recommend that – in addition to the LDL cholesterol or non-HDL cholesterol target – apoB is reduced below 85 mg/dL by treatment.

The European approach was previously more conservative than that of the USA, particularly with respect to primary prevention, but it has recently moved closer. The Fourth Joint Task Force of the European Cardiovascular Societies clearly states that therapeutic targets for serum cholesterol and LDL cholesterol should be below 4.5 mmol/L (175 mg/dL) and below 2.5 mmol/L (100 mg/dL), respectively. Depending on their interpretation of the evidence and their clinical assessment, practitioners are given the option of aiming for a serum cholesterol below 4.0 mmol/L (160 mg/dL) and an LDL cholesterol below 2 mmol/L (80 mg/dL). It is accepted that CHD, peripheral artery disease, cerebrovascular atherosclerotic disease and diabetes call for statin therapy. In primary prevention, people with cholesterol levels at or above 8 mmol/L (320 mg/dL) or LDL cholesterol at or above 6 mmol/L (240 mg/dL) and those with multiple risk factors that place them at a high risk of developing CVD should also receive lipid-lowering medication to achieve these targets.

A new method of assessing cardiovascular (stroke plus CHD) risk has been devised on the basis of collation of data from European interventional trials and epidemiological studies. The only common endpoint for these was cardiovascular death. The studies were conducted using a variety of methods for measuring HDL, with no agreed standardization; HDL has therefore been lost from the predictive equation. The resulting charts, which are called the Systematic Coronary Risk Evaluation (SCORE) charts, show the 10-year risk of cardiovascular death with systolic blood pressure and total serum cholesterol as coordinates. Some versions of the charts replace serum cholesterol with the serum to HDL cholesterol ratio, but these are based on the average HDL cholesterol values for a particular serum cholesterol level. HDL cholesterol is not acting as an independent risk factor.

There are two sets of charts: one for use in countries which have a relatively low risk, such as Belgium, France, Greece, Italy, Luxembourg, Spain and Portugal, and another for all the other countries in Europe. The implication of this is that some factor other than blood pressure, cholesterol and smoking is responsible for geographic differences in cardiovascular risk. Many would disagree with this, concluding that the reason SCORE does not explain differences in rates of CVD in different parts of Europe is because of the omission of HDL cholesterol from the predictive equation and because that equation does not fully take into account blood pressure, cholesterol and smoking. The threshold for being at high risk for fatal CVD is defined as an increase in risk of 5% over the next 10 years, which is equivalent to the threshold of 20% increase in risk of CHD morbidity and mortality over the next 10 years in earlier European guidelines.

The removal of HDL cholesterol from the risk-prediction charts is plainly erroneous. For example, a 60-year-old woman whose serum cholesterol is 8 mmol/L and whose HDL cholesterol is 2 mmol/L (not an uncommon finding) will have a CHD risk that is dramatically different from that of a similarly aged woman with the same serum cholesterol whose HDL cholesterol is only 0.9 mmol/L (see Figure 11.3). Yet both are assigned the same risk by SCORE.

The new European guidelines, like ATPIII and Joint British Societies' (JBS2) (see later), have no charts for assessing risk in diabetes. They assign high cardiovascular risk to diabetes in general. The JBS2 recommendations are based on the Framingham equation for estimating CVD risk (CHD plus stroke morbidity and mortality), which includes HDL cholesterol (Figures 11.2 and 11.3). The JBS2 recommendations

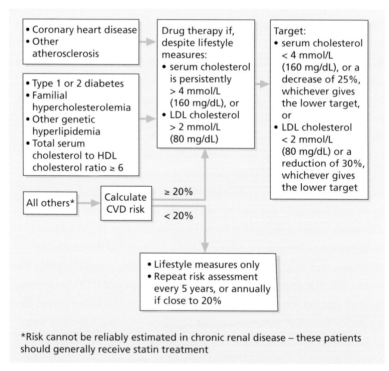

*Risk cannot be reliably estimated in chronic renal disease – these patients should generally receive statin treatment

Figure 11.2 The second Joint British Societies' (JBS2) recommendations for cholesterol-lowering treatment to prevent cardiovascular disease (CVD). Risk of CVD over the next 10 years is estimated using a method based on the Framingham findings, such as the JBS2 chart (Figure 11.3) or the JBS2 computer program (available from www.heartuk.org.uk/HealthProfessionals/ index.php/jbs_cv_risk_assessor). Source: JBS2 guidelines, 2005. LDL, low-density lipoprotein.

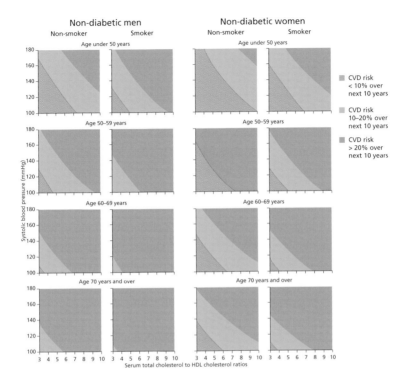

Figure 11.3 Cardiovascular disease (CVD) risk prediction charts for men (left) and women (right) without diabetes. The charts should not be used for calculating risk in people with established coronary heart disease (CHD) (previous myocardial infarction and/or angina), other significant atherosclerosis, left ventricular hypertrophy (on ECG or echocardiography), diabetes or chronic renal disease (decreased glomerular filtration rate and/or proteinuria). Generally, these groups should be considered for lipid-lowering medication in addition to dietary modification if their serum cholesterol is 4 mmol/L (160 mg/dL) or above. The risk estimate should be multiplied by 1.5 in patients with an adverse family history in one first-degree relative (cardiovascular disease or stroke in male first-degree relatives aged < 55 years or a female relative aged < 65 years), and 2 in patients with an adverse family history in two or more first-degree relatives. It should also be multiplied by 1.5 in people who originate from the Indian subcontinent and in impaired fasting glucose (5.6–6.9 mmol/L or 100–125 mg/dL), and by 1.3 in people whose fasting triglyceride level is ≥ 1.7 mmol/L (150 mg/dL). Reproduced with permission from the University of Manchester, UK. These JBS2 charts (2005) have been revised for compatibility with NICE guidance (2008).

129

make a CVD risk of 20% over 10 years the indication for lipid-lowering therapy in primary prevention, if serum cholesterol is persistently 4 mmol/L (160 mg/dL) or higher, or LDL cholesterol is 2 mmol/L (80 mg/dL) or higher.

The recognition that particularly high levels of cholesterol should be treated regardless of estimated risk is also important, because it removes some of the difficulty associated with the diagnosis of FH. The European guidelines, having abandoned HDL cholesterol, set a total serum cholesterol of 8 mmol/L as an indicator for lipid-lowering medication. Certainly this would be absurd in a young woman with an HDL cholesterol of 2 mmol/L or more. The ATPIII guidelines make greater play of LDL cholesterol levels, and a recommendation to treat at an LDL cholesterol level of 4.8 mmol/L (190 mg/dL) or higher with an option to treat at 4.0 mmol/L (160 mg/dL), regardless of calculated risk, takes care of this problem. The JBS2 guidelines make a total cholesterol to HDL cholesterol ratio above 6 an indication for cholesterol-lowering medication.

Although in this book we have provided both the ATPIII scoring system and the British charts for CHD risk assessment, we do not recommend that they be used interchangeably with guidelines for which they were not designed. The risk predicted by the two methods is slightly different, and the thresholds for intervention are therefore specific to the risk-prediction method.

The metabolic syndrome. Both the European recommendations and ATPIII recognize the metabolic syndrome as an indicator of high risk (see Table 7.2 in Chapter 7 for a definition of the metabolic syndrome).

Risk-calculation period. A limitation common to all recommendations based on absolute cardiovascular risk should be noted, namely, how artificial a 10-year span for the calculation of risk can be. Why should a man of 40 with a calculated risk just under that mandating therapy wait until he is 50 before therapy can begin, giving disease 10 more years to develop in his arteries? We know coronary disease has begun by the teens and may be well advanced anatomically by the twenties and thirties. Clinical expression just takes a while longer. The fact of the matter is that our ability to recognize those who are truly at high risk of coronary disease remains very limited, and that is one of the strongest arguments to change the conventional lipid-based diagnostic system. The JBS2 charts currently proposed aim to address some of these concerns by projecting the risk of younger patients forward in time. They are currently available on the website of the Hyperlipidaemia Education and Research Trust UK (www.heartuk.org.uk/HealthProfessionals/index.php/risk_charts). The CVD risk assessor computer program can be downloaded from www.heartuk.org.uk/HealthProfessionals/index.php/jbs_cv_risk_assessor.

Key points – when to treat

- Any clinical evidence of vascular disease is an absolute indication to treat.
- Diabetes mellitus is also an absolute indication to treat.
- Statins are the mainstay of pharmacological therapy.
- Estimation of risk should be broadly based and include age, sex, blood pressure and smoking history, as well as lipid levels and fasting glucose.
- In our opinion, intensive lowering of low-density lipoprotein cholesterol is the principal objective of therapy.

Key references

Barter PJ, Ballantyne CM, Carmena R et al. Apo B versus cholesterol in estimating cardiovascular risk and in guiding therapy: report of the thirty-person/ten-country panel. *J Intern Med* 2006;259:247–58.

British Cardiac Society; British Hypertension Society; Diabetes UK; HEART UK; Primary Care Cardiovascular Society; Stroke Association. JBS 2: Joint British Societies' guidelines on prevention of cardiovascular disease in clinical practice. *Heart* 2005;91(suppl 5): v1–52.

Durrington PN. National and international recommendations for the management of hyperlipidaemia. In: *Hyperlipidaemia: Diagnosis and Management*, 3rd edn. London: Hodder Arnold, 2007:292–309.

Graham I, Atar D, Borch-Johnsen K et al. Fourth Joint Task Force of the European Society of Cardiology and other societies on cardiovascular disease prevention in clinical practice (constituted by representatives of nine societies and by invited experts). European guidelines on cardiovascular disease prevention in clinical practice: executive summary. *Eur J Cardiovasc Prev Rehabil* 2007;14(suppl 2):E1–40.

Grundy SM, Cleeman JI, Merz CN et al. Implications of recent clinical trials for the National Cholesterol Education Program Adult Treatment Panel III Guidelines. *Circulation* 2004;110:227–39.

McElduff P, Jaefarnezhad M, Durrington PN. American, British and European recommendations for statins in the primary prevention of cardiovascular disease applied to British men studied prospectively. *Heart* 2006; 92:1213–18.

McPherson R, Frohlich J, Fodor G, Genest J. Canadian Cardiovascular Society position statement – recommendations for the diagnosis and treatment of dyslipidemia and prevention of cardiovascular disease. *Can J Cardiol* 2006;22:913–27.

National Cholesterol Education Program. Executive summary of the third report of the National Cholesterol Education Program (NCEP) Expert Panel on detection, evaluation and treatment of high blood cholesterol in adults (Adult Treatment Panel III). *JAMA* 2001;285:2486–97.

National Institute for Health and Clinical Excellence. Cardiovascular risk assessment and the modification of blood lipids for the primary and secondary prevention of cardiovascular disease. *Clinical Guideline 67*. London: National Institute for Health and Clinical Excellence, 2008. Available from www.nice.org.uk/CG67

Sniderman AD, Furberg CD, Keech A, Roeters van Lennep JE. Apoproteins versus lipids as indices of coronary risk and as targets for statin treatment. *Lancet* 2003; 361:777–80.

12 Biochemical tests

Methodological sources of variability

Although considerable progress has been made in improving clinical lipid testing, important limitations remain. Only the tests for total cholesterol and apoB and apoAI meet all the requirements described below.

Accuracy describes how closely the results from the particular technique being used in a specific laboratory relate to the results obtained using the accepted reference (or best) method for that variable. That is, how close is the answer in your laboratory to the right answer? All other things being equal, any deviation from the reference method should be systematic. Lack of accuracy, or 'bias', makes comparison of results difficult (if not impossible), and therefore the application of guidelines difficult (if not impossible).

Precision quantifies the difference in repeated measures of the same sample and is expressed as the coefficient of variation (the standard deviation of the repeated measures divided by their average). That is, how variable would the results from the laboratory be if the same sample were measured repeatedly?

Imprecision and inaccuracy should each be less than 3%. Even within these limits, there can be considerable variance in laboratory reports for the same sample, which is why it is recommended to sample more than once before categorizing lipid levels.

Standardization. A test is said to be standardized when all methods that have been approved for routine clinical use yield the same value, because all have been related to an accepted reference. Standardized tests allow results from the same patient, but from different laboratories, to be compared.

Biological sources of variability

These are multiple and can be separated into physiological, behavioral and clinical.

Age, sex and diet are important modifiers of serum lipid levels. Clinical factors also need to be taken into account. For example, lipid levels change abruptly and markedly with many illnesses (e.g. myocardial infarction) and operations (e.g. coronary artery bypass surgery), making accurate diagnosis in the acute setting difficult, if not impossible. Serum cholesterol measured within 24 hours of the onset of chest pain in patients with acute myocardial infarction or coronary insufficiency can be a guide to how high the cholesterol was before the acute event. However, it should never be concluded that a level of less than 5.0 mmol/L (200 mg/dL) measured under these circumstances means that statin therapy is unnecessary. In all patients, subsequent levels should be obtained. Certain medications, including sex steroid hormones, can also affect lipid levels (see Chapter 8).

Total cholesterol

Almost all clinical laboratories now use enzymatic techniques to measure cholesterol, and the measurement is rapid, accurate and easily automated. Non-fasting samples can be used. An abnormally high total cholesterol can occasionally result from either markedly increased high-density lipoprotein (HDL) cholesterol or chylomicrons. With the latter, depending on the level of triglycerides, the risk of pancreatitis may be augmented.

The virtues of total cholesterol measurement are its simplicity and reliability. The drawbacks are that, with the exception of a small minority with markedly high values, there is little difference between the cholesterol levels of those with and those without coronary disease. Moreover, mild or moderate elevation in low-density lipoprotein (LDL) cholesterol with concomitant reduction in HDL cholesterol may result in a normal total cholesterol value.

Triglycerides

Enzymatic methods are also the most commonly used means to measure serum triglycerides. However, these methods are less precise, less accurate and less well standardized. Furthermore, because plasma triglycerides rise markedly after a meal as chylomicron triglycerides enter the plasma, standard practice calls for fasting samples so that, generally, only very-low-density lipoprotein (VLDL) triglycerides will be measured. This imposes considerable difficulty for the patient and considerable uncertainty for the laboratory. Also, many patients with coronary disease have impaired chylomicron clearance from plasma after meals, and the increased remnants may contribute to their risk of vascular disease. This feature is difficult to assess in clinical practice if only fasting samples are taken. However, apoB, whether measured in a fasting or non-fasting state, is frequently elevated in such patients.

LDL cholesterol

LDL cholesterol has become the benchmark laboratory test on which most therapeutic decisions are based. It has many strengths and its value is supported by the epidemiological and therapeutic data gathered over considerable time. Another important advantage is that it is now familiar to physicians the world over. Nevertheless, it has important limitations, and these should not be overlooked.

First, in most laboratories, LDL cholesterol is a calculated value rather than a direct measurement. The usual formulae used are:

- if all concentrations are in mmol/L

$$[\text{LDL cholesterol}] = [\text{total cholesterol}] - \left([\text{HDL cholesterol}] + \left[\frac{\text{triglycerides}}{2.2}\right]\right)$$

- if all concentrations are in mg/dL

$$[\text{LDL cholesterol}] = [\text{total cholesterol}] - \left([\text{HDL cholesterol}] + \left[\frac{\text{triglycerides}}{5}\right]\right).$$

Therefore, all the inaccuracies in each test come into play.

Second, it is not standardized, and therefore values gained using one method are not necessarily the same as those gained using another, making the application of guidelines somewhat imprecise.

Third, just as with total cholesterol, there is so much overlap in the values of LDL cholesterol between those with and those without coronary disease that, unless levels are markedly elevated or very low, it is of little value in determining risk.

Fourth, LDL cholesterol cannot be calculated when triglycerides are above 4.5 mmol/L (400 mg/dL), and major errors can occur once triglycerides are above 2.0 mmol/L (180 mg/dL).

Fifth, the calculation is also frequently in serious error at target levels of LDL cholesterol, that is below 3.0 mmol/L (120 mg/dL).

HDL cholesterol

HDL cholesterol is measured in most clinical laboratories by first precipitating the apoB-containing lipoproteins (VLDL, intermediate-density lipoprotein [IDL] and LDL) and then measuring cholesterol in the supernatant. There is considerable epidemiological evidence demonstrating that the risk of coronary disease is inversely related to the level of HDL cholesterol.

This measurement too has considerable limitations. It is not standardized, and accuracy is particularly critical as there are, in general, only small differences between normal and abnormal levels. Also, it is not clear how a low HDL cholesterol increases the risk of disease. This limitation matters, because a low HDL cholesterol frequently coexists with other abnormalities such as a high triglyceride or high apoB value. Furthermore, there is no pharmacological therapy currently available that increases HDL cholesterol only; thus, no clinical trials have focused on this effect in isolation.

Ratio of total serum cholesterol to HDL cholesterol

This ratio may provide a better approach; it is, for example, the method used in the charts in Figure 11.3, and it includes the risk embodied in LDL cholesterol. There is a wealth of epidemiological data relating to it, and it is therapeutically modifiable by drugs such as statins, albeit because of their effects on LDL cholesterol rather than HDL cholesterol. The ratio also contains, in the HDL cholesterol value, much of the prognostic information contained in triglyceride values, because these are strongly inversely correlated to HDL. It may therefore have an advantage over serum non-HDL cholesterol (serum cholesterol – HDL cholesterol) values, which have also been proposed as overcoming some of the difficulties posed by indirect estimation of LDL cholesterol.

Key points – biochemical tests

- Low-density lipoprotein cholesterol is calculated, not measured, and there are important limitations to its accuracy. Fasting samples are essential.
- Measurement of apoB and apoAI is standardized, and values can be determined from non-fasting samples.
- The ratios of apoB to apoAI and of total cholesterol to high-density lipoprotein cholesterol express the overall risk of disease from dyslipoproteinemia. The ratio of the apolipoproteins is more precise than the ratio of the lipids.

ApoB

Standardized, automated, accurate, inexpensive methods to measure apoB are available. Fasting is not required. There are two forms of apoB: $apoB_{100}$ in VLDL, IDL, LDL and lipoprotein (a) (Lp[a]), and $apoB_{48}$ in chylomicrons and chylomicron remnants. However, even in the peak postprandial hyperlipidemic state, there are so few $apoB_{48}$ particles that fasting is not required. Furthermore, even in hypertriglyceridemic patients, more than 90% of the total apoB particles are LDL particles and therefore total plasma apoB is really determined by LDL apoB.

ApoAI

ApoAI is one of the major apolipoproteins in HDL. It can be accurately and precisely measured using standardized automated assays. There is an inverse correlation with risk, as with HDL cholesterol. There is increasing evidence that apoAI is superior to HDL cholesterol for categorizing risk.

Ratio of apoB to apoAI

This ratio is the apolipoprotein equivalent of the total cholesterol to HDL cholesterol ratio. The AMORIS study, as well as a number of others, has shown the apoB to apoA1 ratio to be superior to the ratio of total cholesterol to HDL cholesterol as a summary index of the risk of vascular disease.

Lp(a)

Lp(a) is measured in only a few laboratories. Considerable work remains to be done in standardizing the assay before it can be introduced widely into clinical practice.

Key references

Contois JH, McConnell JP, Sethi AA et al.; AACC Lipoproteins and Vascular Diseases Division Working Group on Best Practices. Apolipoprotein B and cardiovascular disease risk: position statement from the AACC Lipoproteins and Vascular Diseases Division Working Group on Best Practices. *Clin Chem* 2009;55:407–19.

Rifai N, Warnick GR, Dominiczak MH, eds. *Handbook of Lipoprotein Testing*, 2nd edn. Washington: American Association for Clinical Chemistry Press, 2001.

Useful addresses

American Diabetes Association
1701 North Beauregard Street
Alexandria, VA 22311, USA
Tel: 1 800 342 2383
www.diabetes.org

British Heart Foundation
Greater London House
180 Hampstead Road
London NW1 7AW, UK
Tel: +44 (0)20 7554 0000
www.bhf.org.uk

Canadian Cardiovascular Society
222 Queen Street, Suite 1403
Ottawa, ON K1P 5V9, Canada
Tel: +1 613 569 3407
info@ccs.ca
www.ccs.ca

Diabetes UK
Macleod House, 10 Parkway
London NW1 7AA, UK
Tel: +44 (0)20 7424 1000
info@diabetes.org.uk
www.diabetes.org.uk

European Association for the
Study of Diabetes
Rheindorfer Weg 3
40591 Düsseldorf, Germany
Tel: +49 211 758 4690
www.easd.org

European Atherosclerosis Society
Kronhusgatan 11
SE-411 05, Gothenburg, Sweden
Tel: +46 (0)31 724 27 95
office@eas-society.org
www.eas-society.org

Hyperlipidaemia Education and
Research Trust (H.E.A.R.T) UK
7 North Road, Maidenhead
Berkshire SL6 1PE, UK
Helpline: 0845 450 5988
Tel: +44 (0)1628 777046
ask@heartuk.org.uk
www.heartuk.org.uk

National Cholesterol Education
Program (USA)
www.nhlbi.nih.gov
Third report of the Expert Panel on
Detection, Evaluation, and
Treatment of High Blood
Cholesterol in Adults (Adult
Treatment Panel III)
www.nhlbi.nih.gov/guidelines/
cholesterol/profmats.htm

National Institute for Health and
Clinical Excellence (UK)
www.nice.org.uk

Index

What the reviewers say:

...the sort of publication that anyone willing to take the time to study the condition of epilepsy will gain enormous benefit from. It packs a load of information into just 138 pages and is, at this point in time, easily the most up-to-date book on current antiepileptic drugs

Mike Glynn, President, International Bureau for Epilepsy
on *Fast Facts – Epilepsy*, revised 4th edn, Jan 2010

Brilliant

Dr David Sanders, Chair, BSG Small Bowel and Nutrition Committee
on *Fast Facts – Celiac Disease*, 2nd edn, Sep 2009

The main strengths of the book are the combination of attractive figures and schemes with simple but clear messages in the text...this attractive small book is very useful for general practitioners, non-rheumatologists and allied health professionals

on *Fast Facts – Osteoarthritis*
Rheumatology, Sep 2009

An outstanding up-to-date compilation of facts on psoriasis, a must-read for any healthcare provider with an interest in psoriasis, whether casual or in-depth

Dr Gerald Krueger, Professor of Dermatology, University of Utah School of Medicine,
on *Fast Facts – Psoriasis*, 2nd edn, Jan 2009

This concise, up-to-date, well-illustrated text represents excellent value for money . . . it's unique in being able to pack so much relevant information into such a small volume, which makes it highly readable

British Medical Association,
on *Fast Facts – Minor Surgery*, 2nd edn,
(First Prize, Primary Health Care, BMA Book Awards 2008)

This short textbook provides a quickstop guide to STIs . . . it's handy for both medical students and allied healthcare professionals

British Medical Association,
on *Fast Facts – Sexually Transmitted Infections*, 2nd edn
(Commended, Public Health Care, BMA Book Awards 2008)

www.fastfacts.com

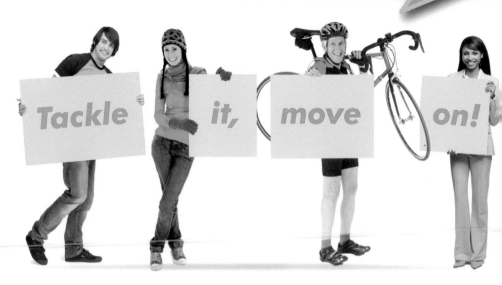